The 7-Day Color Diet

Also by Mindy Weisel:

Daughters of Absence: Transforming a Legacy of Loss
Touching Quiet: Reflections in Solitude
The Rainbow Diet

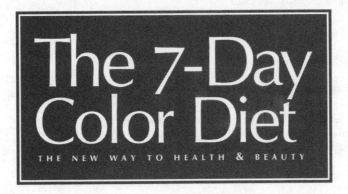

The 7-Day Color Diet

THE NEW WAY TO HEALTH & BEAUTY

M I N D Y   W E I S E L

with her daughters

Carolyn Weisel Miller, M.S., R.D.

Jessica Weisel Courtney, L.E.

CAPITAL
BOOKS, INC.
Sterling, Virginia

Capital Books, Inc.
P.O. Box 605
Herndon, Virginia 20172-0605

ISBN 1-931868-08-5 (alk.paper)

All photos courtesy of Comstock Images, comstock.com, except for the image on page 90 which is from *For the Love of Color*, watercolor, 40" x 60", 2002 by Mindy Weisel.

Illustrations by Mindy Weisel

Library of Congress Cataloging-in-Publication Data

Weisel, Mindy.
The 7-day color diet: the new way to health and beauty/Mindy Weisel, with Carolyn Weisel Miller, Jessica Weisel Courtney; Ariane Weisel, editor.
p. cm.
Includes index.
ISBN 1-931868-08-5
1. Color—Therapeutic use. 2. Color of food. 3. Nutrition. I. Miller, Carolyn Weisel. II. Courtney, Jessica Weisel. III. Weisel, Ariane. IV. Weisel, Mindy. Rainbow diet. V. Title.

RZ414.6.W45 2003
615.8'9—dc21

2002031516

Printed in the United States of America on acid-free paper that meets the American National Standards Institute Z39-48 Standard.

First Edition

10 9 8 7 6 5 4 3 2 1

Always for Shel

contents

foreword

FOREWORD

It has taken an artist to create a truly positive approach to "dieting!" As a dietician I find this ironical, yet somehow logical. When Mindy first asked me to help her with *The Rainbow Diet Book* I was, frankly, reluctant. My training and extensive clinical practice had convinced me that people who needed to lose weight generally have trouble following conventional diets for weight reduction. These diets too often lead to monotony, frustration, and failure.

They do so because they bring about feelings of severe deprivation in the dieter through reductions in portion size, prescribed meal hours, drastic changes in types of foods eaten, and long lists of no-no's. While diets may or may not achieve results, deprivation always takes its toll. The nasty effects of deprivation are all too familiar to most dieters—gnawing boredom or loneliness, food cravings, restlessness, nagging hunger, uncontrolled eating, and subsequent guilt. Over and over again, people go "on" such diets only to later go "off" them.

During the last several years I have had additional training and practice in a new approach to weight management through behavior modification techniques. My patients and students, almost without exception, have had many negative "dieting" experiences. They come to their first classes convinced that food is the root of all their evils—if they could just give it up entirely, their troubles would be ended. It takes many weeks to relearn the simple fact that food is good and beautiful if it is really looked at, appreciated and contemplated, if its aromas are really inhaled, and if its flavors are really savored. Food eaten s-l-o-w-l-y, with ample time for savoring and appreciation, is infinitely more satisfying than food gulped down in guilt. And food that is truly satisfying never leads to feelings of deprivation.

Through her artist's eyes, Mindy Weisel has seen a novel approach to building appreciation of food. The dieter first composes menus with a blank canvas of white foods and, one by one, reintroduces gorgeous colors—first adding red foods, then green, orange, purple, and yellow. The 7-Day Color Diet continually adds foods and dishes as it progresses. It emphasizes long lists of permitted foods and stimulates the jaded chef with recipes. As time goes on, menus become more varied rather than less so. Enhanced appreciation of foods, their appearance, smells, and flavors, invariably results.

Colors tell us a great deal about food on a scientific level, as well as on an artistic one. For example, fruits and vegetables that are good sources of vitamin A are dark yellow or orange (carrots, sweet potatoes, winter squash, cantaloupe, apricots) or dark green (broccoli, green pepper, leaf lettuce, spinach, kale, watercress). Sources of vitamin C (with the exception of cabbage) are colored similarly: yellow lemons, grapefruit, and corn; orange cantaloupe, tangerines, and oranges; red tomatoes and strawberries; green peppers, limes, broccoli, and Brussels sprouts. The B-complex vitamins and iron tend to be bound in brown foods: wheat germ, whole-grain breads and cereals, cooked meats, and liver. For calcium, think of white milk and yogurt and golden cheeses. The rainbow colors have nutritional along with artistic merit!

Mindy's recipe masterpieces, created from her bright palette, are an important part of the 7-Day Color Diet. The titles speak for themselves: "Persian Chicken with Peaches," "Green Bean Crunch," "Veal with Paprika and Pimiento," "Pineapple Squash," "Spanish Orange Fish Fillets," "Red Berries Romanoff." These are delights for all the senses to enjoy.

Where food is concerned, color brings beauty along with nutrition. Two weeks with a rainbow in your kitchen should reawaken your senses to the glories of food and the many joys of eating.

Johanna H. Roth, R.D.,
Bethesda, Maryland
(original consulting nutritionist,
The Rainbow Diet, 1980)

ACKNOWLEDGMENTS

With love and gratitude to my dearest family and friends for their enduring belief in the creative process.

With special thanks to: Ellen Epstein, whose generosity, in directing me to Simon & Schuster, allowed the original *Rainbow Diet Book* to be published twenty-three years ago. And to Madelyn Larsen, my first editor and dear friend.

Noemi Taylor and Anne Louise Bayly, my excellent assistants—who are full of life and genuine caring.

Roy Winkel, my friend and neighbor who so kindly introduced me to Polly Dement. I cannot imagine having been able to complete this book without Polly's excellent guidance to the work being done at the National Cancer Institute.

My publisher and dear friend, Kathleen Hughes, deepest gratitude for her ongoing encouragement, support, and love.

Nancy Sheffner, whose recipes, like our friendship, have withstood the test of time.

Diana My Tran, whose energy creates energy.

Terri Oakley, who has been with us since the first book and helped make everything that followed a reality.

Roz Barak, who opened my eyes to beauty when I was a child and still does.

Beverly and Jack Deutsch, Ron and Rosie Weisel, Bill and Phyllis Weisel, and Elaine and David Beychok, my core.

Debra Freire, co-owner with Jessica of Hydra Skin Care Studio, thank you for continued support and friendship.

Thank you to Sally Aman for all her incredible creative energy.

With deepest love to my father, Amram Deutsch, now a great-grandfather; to Dita Sidlow Deutsch; and to Tobee Weisel, now a great-grandmother, with wishes for their continued positive energy and guidance.

There are now three *new* men in my life since I first wrote The Rainbow Diet Book, who have brought me a world of joy: my sons-in-law Daniel Courtney and David Miller, and my first grandchild, Asher Harris Courtney. We are all grateful for the Courtney and Miller families as well.

And to my husband, Shel Weisel, who is also the father of the three young women with whom I share this book—our daughters Carolyn, Jessica, and Ariane—my love to you always.

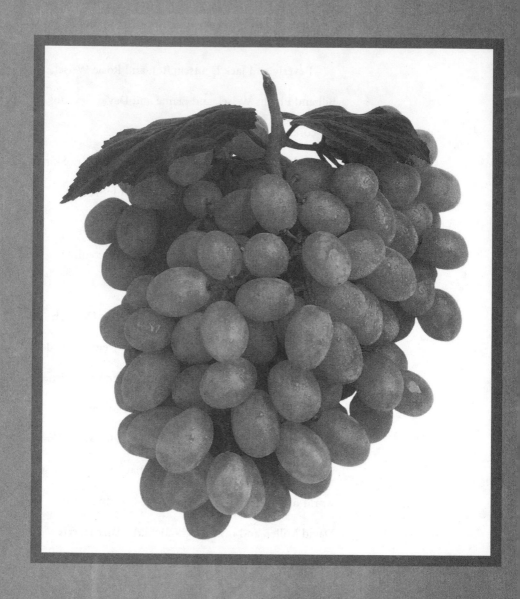

CHAPTER 1

It Took an Artist, a Nutritionist, and an Esthetician to Develop the 7-Day Color Diet

Back in 1980, artist Mindy Weisel opened her paint box and used her extensive knowledge of dieting to develop the "Rainbow Diet." That diet was published in her first book, *The Rainbow Diet Book*. Today she is still slim and healthy and her three daughters have grown up to help her turn that original diet into the full 7-Day Color Diet. Then, as now, Mindy's diet plan is a complete health, eating, and weight loss program based on color control and sound scientific evidence. It is a health-conscious plan that debunks the fads and gets your body in the best shape of your life.

Carolyn Weisel Miller, M.S., R.D., her oldest daughter and a clinical nutritionist, has made sure of that. She reviewed and approved the diet for its nutritional value and added color-coded snacks to keep hunger at bay healthfully. Middle daughter, Jessica

Weisel Courtney, a licensed esthetician, has added seven days of color-coded skin care treatments to help your skin become clearer, healthier, smoother, and more glowing while getting your weight under control and giving your energy a genuine boost. Ariane Weisel, the youngest daughter and an accomplished writer, has added her editing skills to bring all their voices together.

In this chapter, you'll hear each member of the family speak in her own voice. In later chapters, the first-person voice will be that of Mindy.

THE ARTIST'S WAY—A WORD FROM MINDY

You can imagine my absolute amazement when I opened the *Washington Post* in June 2001 to read a headline "Eat Your Purples: Color Coding is the Latest Approach to a Healthful Diet." The article encouraged us to "munch on a rainbow."

The entire following year, articles, books, and scientific journals were surfacing with information touting the health benefits of "colorizing your diet." On May 14, 2002, both the *Washington Post* and the *New York Times* came out with articles, in their health columns, discussing the benefits of paying attention to the colors of the food we eat. As Jane Brody wrote in the *New York*

Times, "Colorize your diet. That is the latest advice from nutrition experts who have studied the health-promoting properties of the vast spectrum of colorful fruits and vegetables now available throughout the country." This was followed by an article in *Newsweek,* in its June 17, 2002, issue, that discussed the latest scientific findings by Tufts University scientists, all of whom have suggested that "research proves the importance of 'pigment power': red, purple and blue pigments are rich in antioxidants, which help prevent cellular damage in humans." Most recently, the National Cancer Institute introduced a marvelous program called "Savor the Spectrum," through which it is educating the public about the inherent health benefits of "eating from the rainbow."

With all this scientific evidence that color plays such a vital role in healthy eating, I decided it was time to reexamine my original Rainbow Diet with the help of my three daughters, now grown into "experts." When *The Rainbow Diet Book* was first published, my daughter Carolyn was eight years old and my daughter Jessica was just three. Ariane wasn't even born yet. Now, twenty-three years later, Carolyn is a clinical nutritionist and a registered dietitian with a master's of science degree, practicing in Manhattan. Jessica is a clinical esthetician and part owner of Hydra Skin Care Studio in Miami. Ariane, a senior at the University of Chicago, is the editor of the University of Chicago Literary Review. It seemed only natural that we collaborate.

The idea for the original *Rainbow Diet Book*, occurred to me one day as I was leaving a drawing class. I had recently given birth to my second daughter, Jessica, and was doing graduate work at America University. I was "feeling fat" at the time, and I seemed to be constantly searching for a diet that would help me shed my unwanted pounds. After class, while collecting my drawing supplies, I noticed another art student, who looked much slimmer than I remembered her. I asked her, naturally, how she had gotten so slim. She told me that for several days she was eating only foods that were orange—cantaloupe, carrots, cheddar cheese, and so on.

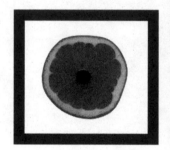

How interesting, I thought. Wouldn't it be a "change" if we just concentrated on the color of foods and not on calories or the amount of carbohydrates? Soon I was imagining days of focusing only on blue foods, red foods, and so on. This idea, almost by itself, grew into a diet based on the variety of natural colors in foods. Rotating the color of foods eaten daily could be a fun way to lose weight, and at the same time, heighten one's awareness of the pleasures of eating a variety of fresh foods. The whole idea appealed to my desire to return to healthy eating instead of the starvation diets to which I had been subjecting myself.

The diet is truly simple. It is fun and colorful and easy and it works. *It works so well you will never have to go on another diet again.* I consider dieting the ultimate punishment. I love eating well. But I also love feeling slim and full of energy. I have been, among other things, a compulsive eater and consequently, I was a compulsive dieter. But most diets amounted to nothing more than miserable acts of deprivation.

The focus in this diet is *not* on counting calories or counting carbograms. This very easy method for losing weight and keeping it off is based on *portion control,* the only true secret about eating right. You learn to enjoy food that is tasty, nutritious, and easily available.

Food can and should taste good and be a source of genuine pleasure. Why feel guilty for eating? Why be afraid of food? Why be confused as to what and how to eat? All this guilt and anxiety over food did not feel right to me. After all, food is supposed to be nourishing, pleasing, and satisfying. Food was put on this earth to take care of us.

Besides, I was tired of counting calories or carbohydrates, living only on protein, and asking everyone I encountered what diet they were on. I couldn't stand my weight going up and down any longer. I wanted to lose my extra weight, learn to eat well, feel good and, hopefully, never diet again.

Over time, I developed my idea into a practical, seven-day program for weight loss. I took the diet and my ideas to Dr. Stuart Seides, a cardiologist at Washington Hospital Center in Washington, D.C. I also discussed the diet with Johanna Roth, a clinical nutritionist in private practice in Washington, D.C. Both Dr. Seides and Mrs. Roth were excited by the idea of a colorful, low-calorie, low-fat eating plan. I immediately put myself on the diet and lost once and for all the extra weight I had been trying to lose. I then collected a test group of people to try the diet. They lost weight and really enjoyed the method. They did not feel deprived or hungry, and they were excited by the variety. All the dieters experienced a heightened awareness of color.

The new 7-Day Color Diet is based on the same principles as other sound diets, but it applies these principles in a way that minimizes the monotony associated with dieting. It focuses on the pleasure that can be derived from eating properly even while you are losing weight.

The diet consists of a *variety* of fruits, vegetables, proteins, and complex carbohydrates (bran cereals, brown rice, brown bread, whole wheat pasta) that supply good tastes, textures, and nutrition. It is easy to stay on this diet because it is interesting, fun, and simple. There is no magic to it, as there is no magic to any diet ever created. It is an eating program that provides energy and satisfaction while you are trying to lose weight. The eating program is clinically proven to give you the ultimate in nutritional content.

In this book there is a weight-loss plan as well as a program for maintaining weight. Menu plans and recipes are provided for everyday use and for entertaining. Life does not have to stop when you are trying to lose weight. You will be able to eat out in any type of restaurant and make wise selections; you will be able to entertain and be entertained, without any stress or strain. Also included in this book is a recommended reading list of good books on the subject of weight loss, good health, and good eating.

It is time for a happy, healthy, and intelligent diet. And for one that works. The 7-Day Color Diet uses color as a control for losing weight. At the same time, it encourages an appreciation for a well-balanced, nutritious, colorful way of eating, which provides a greater chance of staying slim. Unlike most diets, this diet fosters an increased awareness of the beauty of food. By following it carefully, you will definitely lose weight and develop a positive attitude toward eating and staying thin. You will find it possible to enjoy eating and still be healthy and slender throughout your life.

In the appendix we've included the National Cancer Institute's "Savor the Spectrum—5 A Day for Better Health" campaign, intended to educate the public on the nutritional value of various colored fruits and vegetables. Learn more about the foods you'll eat in the 7-Day Color Diet, and the health benefits you'll receive—beyond weight loss. The NCI's research supports the soundness of our diet and emphasizes the importance of the nutritional content in the colors of our food.

> Meals on the diet are easy to prepare. They can be as simple or as elaborate as you choose. The diet will not in any way interfere with your lifestyle. If anything, it should add a great deal of beauty. You can eat out, entertain, feed your family, and use the diet at work.

After a week on this plan, you will feel wonderful, motivated, encouraged, and you will look great! More than that, you will be crafting your body into a natural defense system, ready to fight the toxins that exist in our modern environment, keeping you vigorous for years to come. Enjoy. And to your health.

THE NUTRITIONIST'S WAY —A WORD FROM CAROLYN

My mother has been both an artist and a health nut for as long as I can remember. Her focus on diet and nutrition has contributed to my desire to make a career in the field of nutrition. I remember when she created the original Rainbow Diet back in 1980. It was a natural for someone who loves both color and food. Now that I have become a practicing nutritionist I can attest to the soundness of that original diet, and am honored to collaborate with her in updating it for today.

While we have tried to stay true to the original text, we have made some necessary additions based on nutritional advancements over the years. Besides including brief scientific explanations of the importance of a colorful diet, we've also added a section on soy, and another on complex carbohydrates, "Add a Beige." Additionally, while the focus has always been on portion control as opposed to counting calories as the method for obtaining a healthy weight, we did add some extra servings to each day (compared to the original text) to provide a more healthful approach to weight management.

At the time the original *Rainbow Diet Book* was written, it was widely believed that a restricted calorie diet (900 calories or less per day) was needed to promote healthy weight loss. Today, it is well known that a slower weight loss (one to two pounds per week) on a higher calorie regimen (at least 1,200 to1,500 calories depending on starting weight), in the form of smaller, more frequent meals, is best. This plan helps to spur a continual metabolic calorie burn, while allowing for optimal, yet gradual, weight control.

I once mentioned to my husband over dinner that the more color you have on your plate, the healthier your food is likely to be. He replied, jokingly, "That's funny, I don't remember learning that jelly beans contain any significant nutritive value." What I was referring to, however, is that when it comes to *natural, unprocessed* foods, you can often gauge how healthy your meal is just by the number of brightly colored fruits and vegetables present. Besides making a pretty plate, it has been proven that there are significant nutrients in the colored pigments of these natural foods that host a variety of health-promoting benefits.

Take the tomato, for example. Beneath that glossy red skin lies a *phytonutrient* (a nutrient that is plant derived) called *lycopene.* Lycopene has been shown to reduce the risks of various types of cancers including breast, prostate, and skin cancers. The bluish/purple-pigmented family of fruits and vegetables called *anthocyanins,* which include blueberries, purple grapes, and red cabbage, host powerful antioxidant properties and have also been proven to reduce the risks of heart attacks and diabetes-related complications. *Lutein,* the phytonutrient found in leafy greens, helps to maintain good eyesight. The much talked about phytonutrient *beta-carotene,* located in orange fruits and vegetables such as carrots, sweet potatoes, apricots, and cantaloupe, also boasts powerful antioxidant effects in addition to fortifying the immune system. These benefits, however, are not supplied overnight. It takes years of "colorful dining" to build up these kinds of physiological advantages. (Please refer to the National Cancer

Institute's "Savor the Spectrum" program in the appendix of the book for more complete informational listings.)

Nonetheless, our new 7-Day Color Diet does not attempt to exclude the other food groups. I am a big believer in "everything in moderation," even the jelly bean. Our bodies were built to digest foods from all the various food groups and a calorie is still a calorie no matter what food source it comes from. We must, after all, account for food preferences in our daily diet, lest we feel deprived. More important, however, certain nutrients can only be supplied by specific food groups. Foods from the bread group, for example, which can be rich in fiber, are not necessarily as high in protein as items from the meat group. Servings from the fruit category may be high in vitamin C; items from the milk group, while low in vitamin C, provide some of the best sources of calcium, and so on.

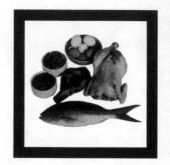

My feeling is that unless one has a known intolerance to a specific food group, all foods should be included equally when planning a healthy diet in order to get the most variety and maximize nutrient consumption. Even the occasional dessert has its place in our diet. That said, given my strong belief in nutrition ·

as preventive medicine, you might as well get the most nutrient density out of everything you put in your mouth, which means choosing healthier options more often than not. Your long-term health depends on it. Enjoy the book, and here's to healthy, colorful eating!

THE ESTHETICIAN'S WAY —A WORD FROM JESSICA

When my artist mother asked me to develop a skin care program to complement the new 7-Day Color Diet, I was intrigued. I had never really considered putting together a full week of beneficial skin treatments based not only on what I know as a licensed esthetician, but also on color. But when I took up this challenge, I realized that color is an inspiring way to organize a week devoted to health and beauty.

Of course, the many fresh fruits and vegetables and low-fat proteins included in the 7-Day Color Diet will do much on their own to make your skin healthier and more beautiful. Just as our bodies benefit from the nutrients and enzymes found in different colored foods and fruits, so does our skin. These enzymes work to give us a brighter, healthier complexion. They also encourage the development of stronger, fresher layers of healthy skin cells. There is so much more we in the skin care business now know as to what can and should keep skin healthy.

Besides a healthy diet, and equally important to clear, healthy glowing skin, is a daily skin care routine. This involves cleansing (geared to whether your skin type is normal, dry, oily, or combination), exfoliating (removing dead skin cells from the surface of the skin), and hydrating (keeping our skin moist and supple). For this reason, and since it should be part of each day, this basic three-part skin routine appears in White Day, just as the 7-Day Color Diet begins with white foods. This White Day treatment should be part of each of the seven days. I'll also give you tips on how to "repair" sun-damaged skin, as well as protect skin from over-exposure to the sun.

After the skin basics of White Day, we add a relax-ing, beneficial skin treatment to go along with the color theme of the day, including recommended products and their application. You'll find some of these prod-ucts right in your refrigerator. Other products I recom-mend to clients at my day spa, Hydra Skin Care Studio in Miami, are included in each treatment. As we add a new color treatment for each day, you'll continue your White Day's cleansing and hydrating routine to receive the full rainbow of benefits.

The seven color treatments will refine, refresh, and relax your skin. The Red Day products, for example, stimulate healthy skin cell production, keeping the skin balanced. The Green Day ingredients allow your skin to heal from harmful toxins that attack it. On Orange and Yellow Days you'll notice a wonderful fresher texture to your skin after using the recommended products, which all provide Vitamin C—an important ingredient that tightens, brightens, and lightens the skin. The Purple Day routine is the ultimate in rejuvenating the skin's surface. Simply and purely, these "rainbow" skin procedures and products will help your skin build up the necessary defenses against aging and the environment. Just as your energy, health, and weight will be at their optimum levels, so will your skin. You will simply glow!

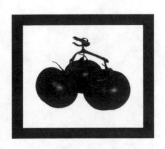

CHAPTER 2

The Beauty of Color Control

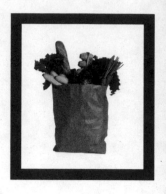

The 7-Day Color Diet is a positive tool that can help you lose weight and keep it off. It will also heighten your awareness and appreciation of the color of the foods you eat. Nothing is more depressing when dieting than facing a bland, colorless meal day after day. No wonder most people have difficulty sticking with diets that deny the sensory delights we expect from food.

The 7-Day Color Diet, on the other hand, is fun, motivating, nutritionally sound, and, best of all, it works. It makes dieting as pleasurable as it can be. It is basically a moderate calorie, moderate carbohydrate diet, based on fresh fruits, vegetables, proteins, and complex carbohydrates. There is a core of white foods in the diet. Most proteins are white, such as chicken, fish, eggs, milk, and cheese. These foods are the staple of the diet. To this basic core, you add fruits and vegetables of different colors on each successive day. For example, on Red Day, the fruit could be a red apple and the vegetable a red tomato. On Green Day, the fruit might be a green pear and you would choose from among the many green vegetables available throughout the year. It is simple to follow. The daily variation of the color of the foods selected provides variety for your eyes and your taste buds. It also serves as your basic eating control.

There are many benefits to this diet. In no way is it monotonous. You will not feel deprived or bored, which means there is a better chance of your staying on it. You won't be busy measuring foods or counting calories all day long. It will deter you from the tendency of thinking how "fattening" each morsel is.

At the same time, it fosters the eating habits and controls that are necessary for any successful weight-loss program. Most important, perhaps, this diet is based on an approach to food meaningful to both the nondieter and dieter. It will help you establish habits and attitudes that will enable you to keep the weight off after you have lost it.

The regimen is based on simple planning and healthy, colorful cooking. All the decisions that normally plague dieters have been made for you. All you have to do is follow the daily diet for the particular color day you are on. Meals on the diet are easy to prepare. They can be as simple or as elaborate as you choose. The diet will not in any way interfere with your lifestyle. If anything, it should add a great deal of beauty. You can eat out, entertain, feed your family, and use the diet at work. There is no magic involved—it is simply a fun way to get slim and stay slim.

The diet begins with White Day, which serves as a sort of "visual fasting." On White Day there is a choice of white proteins—chicken, fish, eggs, cheese or yogurt, and white vegetables and fruits like white grapefruit. The quantity of white vegetables consumed each day is unlimited since they are very, very low in calories and are a good way of filling up without putting on weight.

After White Day, you will discover that the addition of color is in itself a delight. On each successive day, the color of your fruits and vegetables changes. (Your core of white protein choices remains the same daily.) If, however, you find you are very much enjoying a particular color day, you can stay on it until you get bored and, then, go on to the next color day. This method has been particularly successful with people who cook only for themselves and prepare more food than they will

consume in a single day. Each color day provides basically the same quantity of calories and necessary nutrients for healthy dieting. After six days on the diet there
is Rainbow Day, which combines several different colors. You can then start your second week of dieting on
White Day again if you need to or would like to lose
more weight.

Be creative. Experiment mixing your white proteins
and white vegetables with the fruits or vegetables
allowed for each day. One of my favorite quick lunches
is to combine cottage cheese or low-fat yogurt with the
colored fruit or vegetable of the day. Tomatoes and scallions tossed with some cottage cheese and herbs or an
egg-white omelet on Red Day make an entirely different-
tasting meal. You get the idea. Just because you are
eating light does not mean that you have to eat bland.
*Visual blandness is as much of a punishment as blandness
in taste.*

Eat for the right reasons. *Eat because you are hungry. Eat to nourish your body and your senses with good
food.* Learn to eat creatively, and you will lose the
weight you want to and keep it off.

THE SCALE AND WEIGHING YOURSELF

My daughter Carolyn says "the only reason to weigh yourself once a week is for information." It's like getting a bank statement about your body. This business of getting on and off the scale many times a day (or even weighing yourself every morning) is really useless.

Weight fluctuates daily for many reasons, even for something as simple as how much fluid we are retaining. For some people, just seeing a slight rise on the scale ruins their day and then they eat to punish themselves. What is the point of all this? The idea is to feel comfortable and healthy and energetic and attractive. I weigh myself once every three months for "information." I am liberated from the tyranny of the scale and hope you will be too!

FOOD MYTHS
Food Combining

Our stomachs/digestive systems are designed to break down all food groups. There is no scientific evidence whatsoever that there is a need for "food combining"—for example, not eating proteins with carbohydrates. The enzymes are designed to break down, absorb, and use whatever we consume as energy. The idea is to supply ourselves with high-octane fuel, foods that are packed with vitamins, flavor, and are full of nutritional benefits.

Protein Diets

The first few pounds lost on protein diets are due to the immediate loss of water in our bodies. After that the protein becomes a calorie control device. (Look at all the calories you are not taking in by giving up fruits, breads, and complex carbohydrates, but why on earth give up these foods?) The protein is turned into glucose and used for energy as well. Eventually the other nutrients we need are robbed from our muscles to compensate for our not supplying the proper nutrients we require from the many food groups available to us. Also, prolonged protein diets have been proven to cause kidney problems among other ailments. Food is gorgeous, enjoy it!

I would like to add that there is no question that protein keeps us feeling "most full" and helps keep our blood sugar level at its optimum. It is a good idea to have some protein at every meal. But it is not advisable to eat *only* protein. That's torture.

TIPS FOR DIETERS

The following are some positive, helpful tips for dieters.

1.   "Don't go hungry and never build up an urge to overeat," is a phrase to keep in mind always so that blood sugar levels stay even and your metabolism runs at a steady pace. That is one of the key reasons we added a midday snack to the new 7-Day Color Diet.

2.   Eat everything allowed for the day. Never skip a meal. When you skip a meal, you often feel as if you owe yourself something and you end up overeating at the next meal. There is no reason to deprive yourself. Eat regularly, and you will lose the weight once and for all.

3.   Whenever possible, use fresh fruits and vegetables rather than canned or frozen ones. The taste and texture of natural fruits and vegetables, either eaten raw or lightly steamed, are incomparable.

4.   Season food with flavor, not calories. Use fresh herbs, spices, and seasonings when you cook. Go light on the salt, however, as most people with a weight problem have a tendency to retain fluids. It is a good idea to limit your sodium intake.

5.   For added flavor, learn to use fresh lemon juice on your fish, salads, and vegetables. It is also fun to

experiment with good wine vinegars. There is a wide assortment of vinegars available at most markets. Tarragon wine vinegar and garlic wine vinegar are our favorites. Try interesting French mustards as well. There are lemon mustards, mustard with shallots, and mustard with wine. Be creative in your selection of seasonings.

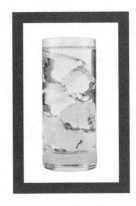

6. Drink six to eight glasses of water daily. Water is very helpful in filling you up and curbing your appetite. Drinking at least six glasses of water is necessary for the proper functioning of the body and is a good habit to incorporate into your daily routine. When you think you are hungry, reach for a glass of water first.

7. Drink decaffeinated coffee and herb tea. Coffee and tea contain caffeine. Caffeine stimulates the body to produce insulin, which may stimulate your appetite. Try to drink no more than one cup of regular coffee a day.

8. Save calories when cooking chicken. Always remove the skin on chicken when preparing any chicken recipe in this book. The skin contains a great deal of fat.

9. Limit your meat meals. We do not recommend eating red meat on this diet, and have not included any recipes containing meat other than chicken or veal. Meat of all kinds, except veal, has a great deal of fat

marbled through it. Most red meats are highly caloric and supply almost double the calories found in chicken or fish. Three ounces of chicken or fish usually supply 150 calories, whereas a three-ounce hamburger or steak contains more than 300 calories. If you cannot live without some red meat in your diet, try to limit it to no more than three meals a week and prepare it as simply as possible.

10. Use a food scale to weigh your protein portions. It will not only help control your portions but it will teach you what a "normal" portion looks like.

11. Weigh yourself only once a week and at the same time of day. Weight fluctuates daily due to fluid retention. It is too discouraging for the dieter to contend with daily fluctuations.

12. Be sure you own excellent cooking utensils. There are a few utensils that we have found to be very good in helping save calories. Nonstick skillets and casseroles are marvelous. They can be sprayed lightly with a variety of natural vegetable sprays on the market today (Pam, Cooking Ease, etc.). A vegetable steamer is another must! The wire vegetable steamer that fits into any pot will always give you a fresh, tasty vegetable with all its vitamins and minerals intact.

13.   Take a multivitamin pill daily.

14.   In case of constipation, add bran. In the unlikely event that constipation should occur, two teaspoons of bran may be added to your daily milk shake.

15.   Do not stay on the 7-Day Color Diet for more than two weeks at a time without your doctor's approval. This diet is not recommended for use during pregnancy, lactation, or childhood.

16.   Be creative. Have fun on this diet. There is a wonderful world of fresh, colorful food for you to enjoy. Use the 7-Day Color Diet recipes for inspiration and good eating, and the Color Beauty Treatments to make your skin glow with health.

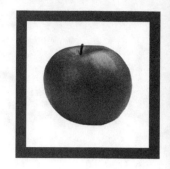

CHAPTER 3

How the 7-Day Color Diet Works

Let's start with some cornerstones of the

7-Day Color Diet.

THE COLOR DIET BREAKFAST: WHAT WE NOW CALL "SMOOTHIES"

When I designed the original Rainbow Diet breakfast,

so many years ago, who knew what I then called a "milk

shake" would turn into what we now call "smoothies."

I have added one tablespoon of protein powder to the

original recipe for an extra morning boost.

The 7-Day Color Diet breakfast consists of nonfat

milk and fruit whipped up in a blender with ice for a

thick, rich milk shake. The milk shake is packed with

protein and will provide energy, vitamins, and minerals

throughout the entire morning. It is also wonderful

when dieting to have something thick, creamy, and

filling for breakfast.

The milk shake is very easy to prepare. By adding

fruit of the particular color day you are on, you can

vary the taste. On Red Day, for example, you can have a

strawberry milk shake, and on Yellow Day, you can make either a banana or pineapple milk shake.

The basic milk shake recipe is one of the following:

Either 1 cup nonfat milk (lactose-free nonfat milk
    or vanilla-flavored soy milk is great too if regular
    milk does not agree with you), or 1 cup nonfat
    yogurt or $1/2$ cup tofu (silken) combined with
    $1/2$ cup nonfat milk
Add: 1 tablespoon protein powder
1 cup color fruit of the day (colored fruit lists are
    located at the beginning of each color chapter)
1 teaspoon vanilla extract
1 tablespoon honey or artificial sweetener to taste
6 to 8 ice cubes

This is all whipped up in the blender or food processor for one to two minutes until thick and creamy. To this basic recipe you can add any fruit of the color day you are on, or you can have the milk shake and fruit separately. On Orange Day, I prefer to eat the orange separately and add one teaspoon instant coffee to the basic milk shake to make a java-flavored shake. It's delicious!

The main point to remember about breakfast is to make sure you have milk and fruit at that time. This is a wonderful combination of foods to get you going for the day and to keep you from being hungry. It provides a great deal of energy, and you will not feel like you are dieting.

ADD A BEIGE—CARBOHYDRATES

Carbohydrates are often viewed as the villain of the

dieting world. It is well known, however, that without carbohydrates a healthy diet is not possible. Complex carbohydrates, which include whole grain breads, cereals, and legumes, provide unending health benefits. Despite their neutral color, when used in moderation and in conjunction with other healthy foods, carbohydrates provide the best way to round out the diet rainbow. Abundant in B vitamins and rich in fiber, complex carbohydrates can prevent certain types of cancers and promote a healthy digestive tract. Without sufficient intake of carbohydrates, which are broken down into glucose as the preferred source of fuel for our bodies and brains, we start to metabolize other nutrients for fuel, and that can wreak havoc on our bones, muscles, and other vital organs.

These complex carbohydrates may be added at breakfast or lunch:

1 slice bread (rye, wheat, or pumpernickel)
1 cup cereal (high fiber—low fat: i.e., oatmeal, All-Bran, Go Lean, or Bran Flakes)
1 English muffin (whole wheat)
1 small whole wheat pita bread
2 rye crisp crackers, 2 rice cakes, or 3 melba toasts
1 cup brown rice
1 cup whole wheat pasta
1 small baked potato
1 ounce oat bran pretzels

THE PROTEIN LIST

Throughout the 7-Day Color Diet, you'll be asked to choose one portion per meal from the following Protein List.

- One 4-ounce serving of protein from the recipes in each Color Day
- One 4-ounce serving of fish, chicken, turkey, *or* tofu
- 1 cup of cottage cheese (lowfat)
- 2 eggs (limit to 4 per week) or 5 egg whites
- 2 ounces of hard cheese (lowfat)
- 1 cup nonfat or low-fat yogurt (may also be used in soups, dressings, or desserts)
- 1 tablespoon of peanut butter

FOR VEGETARIANS

The "color" white is used as the protein base for the color-coded recipes in the 7-Day Color Diet. For those of you who do not eat chicken, fish, eggs, cheese, and milk, soy is another "great white way" for you to add protein to your meal. Soy, found in soy milk, tofu, soybeans, and soybean oil, among other products, has also been touted in recent years as having tremendous health benefits. Aside from aiding in menopausal symptoms, soy also helps to reduce the risks of certain types of cancers and heart disease. Soy has also been shown to reduce the risk of osteoporosis, especially significant for vegetarians who do not eat products from the milk group.

SOY PROTEIN: WHY AND HOW TO USE IT

For those interested in increasing soy in their diets, the following foods can be substituted in the daily diet, as well as in any of the recipes: soy burgers instead of chicken or fish; soy milk instead of regular milk or yogurt. One and one-half tablespoons of soy protein powder can be substituted, instead of milk, for the morning milk shake, or added to soups, salad dressings, or brown rice as a protein supplement. Soy protein can be found in any good health food store. A variety of products are available at the supermarket, everything from soy-based, vegetarian "burgers," "chicken patties," and "hot dogs" to "stuffed cabbage." They are delicious, low-fat, and add a great deal of variety.

Adding soy to your diet is highly beneficial. Soy provides photochemicals known as isoflavones. These isoflavones, made up of genistein and daidzein, mimic the way estrogen is used in the body. For example, women in Asia, where the diet is high in soy products, have fewer menopausal symptoms than women in America. Hot flashes and mood swings are foreign to

For those interested in increasing soy in their diets, the following foods can be substituted in the daily diet, as well as in any of the recipes: soy burgers instead of chicken or fish; soy milk instead of regular milk or yogurt. One and one-half tablespoons of soy protein powder can be substituted, instead of milk, for the morning milk shake, or added to soups, salad dressings, or brown rice as a protein supplement.

them. Because of soy protein's amino acid composition, soy protein can keep insulin levels steadier, which then helps control heart disease, diabetes, and certain types of cancer. When I wrote *The Rainbow Diet Book*, twenty-three years ago, soy products were hard to come by, but now every supermarket in the country carries soy burgers in their freezer sections and soy milk and soy cheese, yogurts, and tofu in their regular refrigerator sections. I encourage you to explore if you haven't already. Adding soy protein is a great boost to our energy and all-around good health.

THE 7-DAY COLOR DIET PLAN

Now you are ready to learn how to put all the colorful elements of the diet together. The basic plan is as follows. More complicated menus appear at the beginning of each Color Day.

Sample Menu

Breakfast
1 fruit milk shake or "smoothie" (color of the day)
Add a Beige or an extra fruit serving

Lunch
Small salad or small cup of soup (from the appropriate Color Day chapter)
One 4-ounce serving of protein from the Protein List

Add a Beige

Unlimited vegetables (color of the day)

1 fruit (color of the day)

Beverage (coffee, tea, or diet soda)

Snack

Add a Beige or 1 fruit (color of the day)

Half of a 4-ounce protein serving from the Protein List

Dinner

One 4-ounce serving of protein from the Protein List

Unlimited vegetables (color of the day)

Add a Beige

1 fruit (color of the day) or 4 ounces of sorbet (based on color of the day)

Beverage (coffee, tea, or diet soda)

Staying hydrated is key so always remember that the "beverage" can be water, water, water!

Additional Daily Allowances:

1 tablespoon butter, mayonnaise, margarine, or 2 tablespoons olive oil (may be used in cooking or on salads)

Unlimited herbs, wine vinegar, rice vinegar, lemon juice, mustard, spices

Herb tea, decaffeinated coffee, diet soda

Sugar-free gelatin

Unlimited white vegetables (mushrooms, cauliflower, bean sprouts, white cabbage, endive)

Sugar-free Popsicles and Fudgesicles (limit to 1 per day)

Sugarless gum

Skim milk added to coffee (limit to 1 cup total per day)

In the next chapters you'll find out how to follow the diet through each Color Day, along with delicious, easy-to-prepare recipes. To get you started, here are a list of color-coded foods and a sample menu for each day. There is an asterisk after the names of those items for which a recipe appears in the appropriate Color Day.

Please note: The recipes vary in serving sizes, as some are easy to prepare in large quantity, either to have on hand all week or to serve to a large group when entertaining. Be sure you stick to the portions recommended.

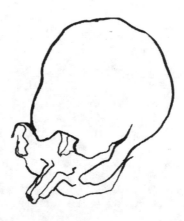

This is Day One of your colorful new way of eating. It is your day of "visual fasting." After White Day, you'll be adding glorious color after color, as you lose pound after pound. Here is the basic plan for this day. Remember, tofu can be substituted for chicken, fish, or meat in any recipe—especially for those who are vegetarian and need extra protein and/or calcium at a particular meal. A recipe is included for each dish marked with an asterisk. Let's start with the foods you can eat today.

day 1 white

white day sample menu

Breakfast

    Grapefruit

    Vanilla Honey Milk Shake*

    Coffee or tea

Lunch

    Mushroom and Endive Salad with Herb Vinaigrette*

    5-egg-white omelette

    Whole wheat bread, 1 slice

    Herb tea

Snack

    4 ounces nonfat vanilla yogurt

    2 salted rice cakes

Dinner

    1 cup Russian Mushroom Soup*

    White Garlic Chicken, 4 ounces*

    Steamed Cauliflower with Herbs

    Cinnamon Broiled Grapefruit, $1/2$*

    Decaffeinated coffee or herb tea

white foods list

White Fruit:
White grapefruit

White Vegetables:
Unlimited amounts of mushrooms, onions, cabbage, cauliflower, endive, bean sprouts, alfalfa sprouts, pattypan squash, water chestnuts

WHITE DAY RECIPES

White Salads and Luncheon Dishes

COLD CAULIFLOWER SALAD

3 heads cauliflower
3 cups plain nonfat yogurt
4 tablespoons Dijon mustard
2 teaspoons salt
1 teaspoon freshly ground pepper
1/2 cup chopped, fresh parsley

Break cauliflower into small florets. Cook in boiling water for 5 to10 minutes. Do not overcook. Vegetables should be crisp. Blanch in cold water. Drain. Combine all ingredients except parsley and pour dressing over cauliflower until well coated. Chill. Before serving, toss chopped, fresh parsley into salad.

MUSHROOM AND ENDIVE SALAD
WITH HERB VINAIGRETTE

1/2 cup mushrooms, sliced
1/2 cup bean sprouts
1 small endive, sliced

Combine vegetables in large salad bowl. Top with 2 tablespoons Herb Vinaigrette.

Remember that recipes make more than one serving unless otherwise specified. Use the recommended serving size from the Basic Color Diet found in the previous chapter.

WHITE DAY LUNCHEON SALAD WITH VINAIGRETTE DRESSING

1 cup shredded white cabbage
1/2 cup shredded low-fat Swiss cheese
1/2 teaspoon caraway seed
1/4 cup Vinaigrette Dressing
Crisp lettuce leaves
1 hard-cooked egg

Mix cabbage and cheese. Combine caraway seed with vinaigrette. Pour over cabbage and cheese. Let marinate several hours. Serve on crisp lettuce and top with crumbled hard-cooked egg.

Vinaigrette Dressing

1 tablespoon vinegar
2 tablespoons oil
1 clove garlic, crushed
1 teaspoon Dijon mustard
1 teaspoon salt
1/2 teaspoon freshly ground pepper

Herb Vinaigrette

2 tablespoons wine vinegar
1 teaspoon Dijon mustard
1/2 teaspoon salt
1 clove garlic, mashed
3 tablespoons minced herbs (parsley, dill, tarragon)
4 tablespoons olive oil

Blend all ingredients together until smooth.
Makes 3/4 cup of dressing.

White Soup

RUSSIAN MUSHROOM SOUP

$^1/_2$ pound mushrooms
1 tablespoon olive oil
$^1/_2$ teaspoon caraway seed
$^1/_2$ teaspoon imported paprika
$3^1/_2$ cups chicken stock
1 teaspoon dried dill, or 2 teaspoons fresh
Salt and pepper to taste

Wash mushrooms quickly, dry thoroughly, and slice.
Melt olive oil in a nonstick saucepan and sauté mushrooms, caraway seed, and paprika for 1 minute. Add
chicken stock and simmer, covered, for 30 minutes.
Add dill. Taste for seasoning. Whisk to mix thoroughly
and serve.

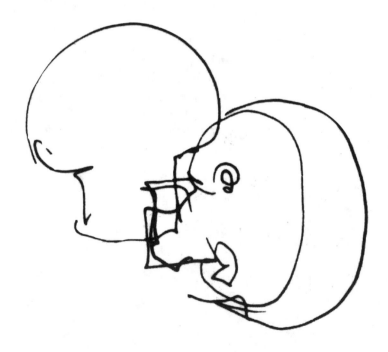

White Protein Dishes

WHITE SALAD WITH ITALIAN TUNA DRESSING

1 cup cottage cheese
1 hard-boiled egg
1 can tuna, 3 1/2 ounces, packed in water
1 tablespoon lemon juice
1 clove garlic, mashed
1/4 small white onion, chopped
Salt and freshly ground pepper

Puree cottage cheese in blender until smooth. Add egg, tuna, lemon juice, garlic, and onion and blend until smooth. Season with salt and pepper to taste. Pour dressing over large salad of raw white vegetables (sliced mushrooms, cauliflower, endive, bean sprouts, and shredded cabbage) and serve as a full luncheon meal.

WHITE MUSHROOM FISH BAKE

1 1/2 tablespoons olive oil
2 tablespoons finely minced shallots or scallions
1 cup thinly sliced mushrooms
2 1/2 pounds fish fillets (flounder, sole, or haddock)
Salt and white pepper
2/3 cup dry white wine

Preheat oven to 350 degrees. Smear half the olive oil in a baking-serving dish. Sprinkle with half the shallots and mushrooms. Place the fish fillets on top of the mushrooms and shallots. Season fish with salt and pepper. Top with remaining shallots and mushrooms. Pour in the wine. Top with remaining olive oil. Bake for 20 minutes. Do not overcook.

WHITE DAY HERB BROILED FISH

2 pounds fish steaks (halibut, haddock, or cod)
2 tablespoons melted butter
1/2 small onion, grated
2 tablespoons lemon juice
1 teaspoon salt
1/4 teaspoon pepper
1/4 teaspoon marjoram
2 tablespoons chopped fresh parsley

Put fish on broiler rack (or use disposable broiling pans). Mix butter, onion, lemon juice, salt, pepper, marjoram, and parsley and pour half over fish. Broil on one side (10 minutes) until done. Turn fish, add remaining sauce, and broil another10 minutes.

WHITE GARLIC CHICKEN

Delicious!

1 chicken, cut into serving pieces
1 teaspoon salt
1/2 teaspoon pepper
1/2 cup wine vinegar
4 cloves garlic, finely minced

Preheat oven to 350 degrees. Place chicken in roasting pan. Season with salt and pepper. Pour vinegar and sprinkle garlic on top. Bake uncovered for 40 minutes. Preheat broiler. Put chicken under broiler for 10 to15 minutes until all pieces are crisp. Brush chicken with gravy while broiling.

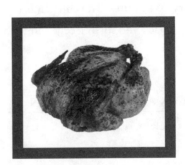

ROAST CHICKEN WITH HERBS

If you don't feel like roasting a whole chicken but have 4 pounds of chicken pieces, you can mix the lemon juice, herbs, and minced onion and coat each piece with this mixture. Roast in roasting pan until done.

1 4-pound roasting chicken
1/2 lemon
Salt and freshly ground black pepper
1 small onion
1/2 teaspoon dried thyme
1 bay leaf
1/2 teaspoon dried tarragon
1 large sprig fresh parsley

Preheat oven to 350 degrees. Rub inside of chicken with half a lemon and sprinkle with salt and pepper. Add a small onion to the cavity with the herbs. Truss and place the chicken in a roasting pan. Roast for 1 1/2 hours, basting every 20 minutes. The chicken is done when the leg moves back and forth freely and the juices run clear yellow.

WHITE DAY MARINATED CHICKEN

1 4-pound chicken, quartered

Marinade
1/2 cup dry white wine
2 cloves garlic, minced
1 large onion, coarsely chopped
1 teaspoon rosemary
1/2 teaspoon salt
1/2 teaspoon freshly ground black pepper
1/2 teaspoon paprika

Mix marinade ingredients well. Pour over chicken. Marinate chicken in glass bowl, covered, in refrigerator. Turn pieces once. Barbecue or broil, basting with marinade.

White Vegetables

CAULIFLOWER CURRY

1 teaspoon olive oil
1 teaspoon cumin seed
1 teaspoon mustard seed
1 clove garlic, minced
$1/2$ teaspoon freshly ground pepper
1 tablespoon curry powder
8 ounces extra-firm tofu, cut into cubes
4 cups cut-up cauliflower
$1/4$ cup vegetable stock

Heat oil in large sauté pan over medium heat. Add next 5 ingredients and sauté for 1 minute. Add tofu, cauliflower, and vegetable stock. Cook, stirring occasionally, for 15 minutes or until cauliflower is tender. Serve hot or cold. Serves 4.

STEAMED CAULIFLOWER WITH HERBS

Excellent filling, low-calorie vegetable to have with fish or chicken.

1 large head cauliflower
2 cups water
$1/2$ cup minced fresh herbs
Salt and pepper to taste

In large pot with vegetable steamer inserted, bring water to a boil. Break cauliflower into florets and place in steamer. Steam for 20 minutes. Refresh cauliflower under cold water and toss with fresh herbs (parsley, dill, tarragon) and seasoning.

MUSHROOMS À LA GRECQUE

This court bouillon, or simmering broth, is a good way to cook low-calorie vegetables such as celery, eggplant, and green peppers. The vegetables gain in flavor as they marinate in the broth and can be eaten cold in a salad or as an hors d'oeuvre at any time.

1 pound fresh mushrooms
2$\frac{1}{2}$ cups simmering court bouillon

Court Bouillon

2 cups water
$\frac{1}{3}$ cup lemon juice
1 tablespoon oil
$\frac{1}{2}$ teaspoon oil
2 tablespoons minced shallots or scallions
6 sprigs parsley
1 small celery stalk with leaves
$\frac{1}{4}$ teaspoon fennel seed
$\frac{1}{4}$ teaspoon thyme, dried
12 peppercorns

Place all ingredients for the court bouillon in a 2$\frac{1}{2}$-quart saucepan and simmer, covered, for 10 minutes. Wash mushrooms quickly, dry thoroughly, and slice. Add mushrooms to broth and simmer 10 minutes. Remove mushrooms and set aside. Boil down the court bouillon until reduced to about $\frac{1}{3}$ cup. Season with salt and pepper. Strain broth over mushrooms. The mushrooms may be covered and refrigerated for 3 days.

beauty

WHITE DAY BEAUTY TREATMENT
A Day of Cleansing and Hydrating

White Day is a day of cleansing and purifying. It is the day when you begin to appreciate that a balanced skin care routine will not only give you a healthy complexion, it will also help protect you from skin cancer and provide anti-aging benefits. White Day is the basis for this entire skin care program.

How you cleanse, hydrate, and protect your skin from harmful UVA/UVB sun rays depends upon your skin type: normal/combination, dry/sensitive, or oily.

For normal/combination skin, cleansing is simple. This skin type tends to be "even" in tone and texture, with small- to medium-sized pores. It is called "combination," however, because many "normal" complexions have what is called the "t-zone"—the area of skin on the forehead and around the nose and chin. The oil glands in this area are more active and tend to increase oil production, causing slightly larger pores.

If your skin is normal or a combination skin type, use a soap-free cleanser both morning and night, and rinse it off with lukewarm water. Always use a soap-free product because soap strips the skin of its natural lipid barrier and causes irritation that increases the rate at which the skin ages. Cleansing is important not only to remove dirt, but also to slough off the dead cells that sit on the skin's surface, so that healthy new cells can be produced. After cleansing, it is vital to hydrate your skin to prevent wrinkling. Use a product that provides enough moisture without weighing your skin down with unnecessary oils, such as Dermalogica Special Cleansing Gel and Dermalogica Active Moist for normal skin.

Dry/sensitive skin needs extra special care. Gently cleanse to remove dirt and dead skin cells with an emulsion that has both oil and water. Dry/sensitive skin tends to have small pores and a dehydrated surface layer, making it feel "tight" and "worn looking." Many factors may cause this sensitivity, including the environment and using the wrong products. Sensitive skin can appear red and scaly, with dry patches around different areas of the face. A rich moisturizer used morning and night, after cleansing, will help. I recommend Dermalogica Ultra Calming Cleanser and Dermalogical Intensive Moisture Repair for dry skin.

An oily skin condition is the result of overactive oil glands that produce an excessive amount of oil in the skin. With oily skin, the pores are large and have a shiny appearance. Cleansing should be done with an oil-free—as well as soap-free—cleanser that will remove the daily buildup of oil and dirt on the surface of the skin. I recommend Dermalogica Dermal Clay Cleanser and Dermalogica Oil Control Lotion for oily skin.

No matter what your skin type, drink at least eight glasses of water a day to hydrate your skin from the inside and rid the body of the buildup of toxins that clog your pores.

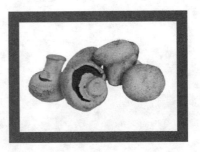

From the visual fasting of White Day, we move into the most exciting of all colors—red. But don't get carried away. Keep your portions under control while you relish the flavors of these sensual red foods.

dayTWO

day 2 | red

Red Day Sample Menu

Breakfast

Strawberry Milk Shake*

1 slice rye toast

Coffee or tea

Lunch

Cold Cauliflower Salad with Yogurt Dill Dressing*

Stuffed Tomato, 1*

Whole wheat bread, 1 slice

Herb tea

Snack

4 ounces nonfat strawberry yogurt

1 ounce oat bran pretzels

Dinner

Iced Tomato Soup, 1 cup*

Veal Scallops Marinara, 4 ounces*

Steamed Cauliflower with Herbs*

Red Day Baked Apple, 1*

Decaffeinated coffee

Red Foods List

Red Fruits:
1 cup strawberries,
1 apple,
1 cup raspberries,
1 cup watermelon

Red Juices:
6 ounces tomato juice
or 6 ounces V-8 juice

Red Vegetables:
1 tomato; unlimited
amounts of red
cabbage, radishes,
pimientos, red peppers

RED DAY RECIPES
Red Salads and Luncheon Dishes

RED DAY TUNA-APPLE SALAD

1 can solid white tuna, packed in water
1 red apple, unpeeled, cored,
   and chopped in large pieces
2 teaspoons lemon juice
1 rib celery, thinly sliced
1 white scallion, thinly sliced

Dressing
1/3 cup plain low-fat yogurt
1 tablespoon mayonnaise
1/2 teaspoon curry powder
1/4 teaspoon salt
1/4 teaspoon white pepper

Break tuna up in salad bowl. Pour lemon juice over apples to keep white. Add apples, celery, and scallion to tuna and toss well. Mix dressing and pour over tuna-apple salad. Toss well. Chill 1 to 2 hours. Serve on bed of salad greens.

STUFFED TOMATOES

Quick luncheon dish. You can use 1 cup tuna or cottage cheese instead of the eggs.

2 large tomatoes
4 hard-boiled eggs, finely chopped,
   or 6 boiled egg whites
1 scallion, minced
2 tablespoons minced fresh parsley
1 tablespoon mayonnaise
Salt and pepper to taste
Pulp of tomato, coarsely chopped

Cut tomato tops off. With sharp knife cut out the pulp and set aside, leaving a tomato shell with a deep cavity. Turn tomato shells over on a paper towel and let drain for 30 minutes. Combine chopped egg, scallion, parsley, mayonnaise, salt, pepper, and coarsely chopped tomato. Spoon into tomato shells. Serve on a bed of lettuce.

COTTAGE CHEESE PIMIENTO SALAD

$1/2$ cup large, sliced pimientos
   or 1 sweet red pepper, roasted, cut into strips
$1\,1/2$ cups cottage cheese
1 cup bean sprouts
1 teaspoon salt
1 teaspoon pepper

Toss ingredients together for a delicious, quick lunch. Fresh, minced herbs can be added before serving. To roast your own peppers: Put peppers on an aluminum foil sheet and bake 20 minutes at 350 degrees.

RED DAY SALAD DRESSING

*The following salad dressing may be poured over
unlimited white vegetables for a filling, low-calorie salad.*

8 ounces V-8 juice
1 tablespoon salad oil
2 teaspoons seasoned salt (Vegit if available)
2 teaspoons freshly ground pepper
1 teaspoon dill
1/4 teaspoon Tabasco sauce
1 clove garlic, minced

Whisk all ingredients together and chill until
ready to serve.

Red Soups

RED DAY GAZPACHO

2 large, ripe tomatoes, chopped
1 small onion
1/2 clove garlic
1/2 long, red chili pepper
2 cups tomato juice
1/4 cup white wine vinegar
2 teaspoons olive oil
1/4 cup dry white wine
1 teaspoon paprika
1/4 teaspoon cumin
Salt, pepper, Tabasco sauce to taste
1/2 teaspoon Worcestershire sauce

Put all ingredients in a blender or food processor and
puree until smooth. Strain. Chill several hours.

HOT CURRIED TOMATO SOUP

Good luncheon dish on a cold day.

3 cups tomato juice
3 cups chicken broth
2 teaspoons lemon juice
1 teaspoon sugar substitute
4 whole cloves, tied in cheesecloth
1/2 teaspoon imported curry powder, or to taste
Salt
Dash of Tabasco sauce
4 tablespoons grated Jack cheese

Combine tomato juice and chicken broth. Bring to a boil. Reduce heat. Add lemon juice, sugar substitute, and cloves. Add curry powder and stir. Season with salt and Tabasco sauce to taste. Heat thoroughly for 5 to 10 minutes. Remove the cloves. Pour into mugs and garnish each with a tablespoon of Jack cheese.

ICED TOMATO SOUP

1 1/2 cups plain low-fat yogurt
3 cups tomato juice
1 tablespoon lemon juice
1 scallion, minced
1 clove garlic
1 teaspoon curry powder
1/2 cup fresh dill, or 1 tablespoon dried
3 tablespoons chopped, fresh parsley
Salt, pepper, and a dash of Tabasco sauce to taste
Chopped cucumber and fresh parsley

In blender or food processor blend yogurt until smooth. Add tomato juice, lemon juice, scallion, garlic, curry, dill, and parsley. Blend well. Season with salt and pepper to taste. Add 1 or 2 drops of Tabasco sauce. Garnish individual soup bowls with cucumber and parsley. Serve well chilled.

Red Protein Dishes

RED DAY SOLE PROVENÇAL

Delicious hot or cold.

1 small onion, chopped
2 large ribs of celery, chopped
1 tablespoon oil
1 16-ounce can tomatoes
2 tablespoons parsley
2 bay leaves
1 1/2 teaspoons salt
1/2 teaspoon pepper
1/2 cup dry white wine
1 pound fillet of sole

Sauté onions and celery in oil until tender. Add tomatoes, parsley, bay leaves, salt, pepper, and wine. Cover and simmer for 20 minutes. Add fish and simmer, covered, for 15 minutes longer.

FRENCH FISH STEAKS

These are delicious!

4 halibut steaks, 1 inch thick
Salt, white pepper, and paprika
1 tablespoon butter
1/2 pound mushrooms, thinly sliced
1 onion, finely minced
1 clove garlic, finely minced
2 tablespoons chopped parsley
1 16-ounce can stewed tomatoes

Preheat oven to 350 degrees. In nonstick baking pan, place halibut steaks and season well with salt, white pepper, and paprika. In nonstick saucepan sauté mushrooms, onion, and garlic in butter until soft. Add parsley and tomatoes and heat through. Spoon sauce over fish steaks and bake, uncovered, for 30 to 40 minutes.

HUNGARIAN BAKED FISH

1 large onion, sliced
1 pound fresh fish fillets
1 teaspoon salt
1/2 teaspoon pepper
2 tablespoons Hungarian paprika
2 tablespoons fresh dill, or 1 teaspoon dried
2 large tomatoes, coarsely chopped
1/2 cup white wine

Preheat oven to 350 degrees. In a nonstick casserole make a bed of the onion slices. Lay fish fillets flat on top of onions. Season fish with salt, pepper, paprika, and dill. Pour chopped tomatoes and wine over all. Bake covered for 30 to 40 minutes. Baste once or twice.

GRILLED SALMON STEAKS

4 salmon steaks
3 tablespoons chopped, fresh dill
3 tablespoons lemon juice

Preheat broiler. Rub salmon steaks with dill and lemon juice. Put on broiling pan and broil for 10 minutes on each side. Season with salt and pepper.

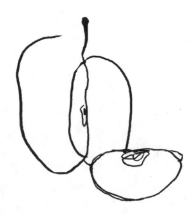

CHICKEN PAPRIKA

1 large onion, minced
1/2 pound mushrooms, sliced
1 tablespoon olive oil
1 chicken, cut into quarters
1 clove garlic, peeled
2 teaspoons salt
1 teaspoon pepper
2 tablespoons imported paprika
2 teaspoons dried basil, crushed
1/2 teaspoon oregano
1/2 teaspoon rosemary (optional)

Preheat oven to 350 degrees. Sauté onion and mushrooms in oil. Rub chicken with fresh garlic and season with salt, pepper, paprika, basil, oregano, and rosemary. Place chicken pieces in casserole and cover with onions and mushrooms. Bake covered for 45 minutes and uncovered for 30 minutes. Baste several times while chicken is baking.

PODVARAK CHICKEN AND SAUERKRAUT

The recipe for this delicious Viennese chicken dish was given to me by one of my dearest friends, Vera Loeffler.

2 pounds sauerkraut
3 pounds chicken, cut into serving pieces
Salt
2 tablespoons oil
1/2 cup finely chopped onions
1/2 teaspoon finely chopped garlic
1 tablespoon finely chopped hot chili peppers
Freshly ground black pepper
1/2 cup chicken stock

Wash sauerkraut under cold, running water and soak in cold water for 20 minutes more to reduce sourness. Squeeze it dry by the handful. Salt chicken pieces generously. Brown chicken well in nonstick skillet using 1 tablespoon oil. As each piece browns, remove to a platter until all the chicken is done. Set aside. In the same skillet, heat the other tablespoon of oil and sauté onions and garlic until slightly translucent. Add the sauerkraut, chili peppers, and a few grindings of black pepper. Cook uncovered for 10 minutes over medium heat. Using tongs lay chicken pieces on top of sauerkraut. Pour chicken stock over chicken. Bring the liquid to a boil. Reduce heat to low. Cook, covered, for 45 minutes or until chicken is tender. Serve the sauerkraut on a platter with the chicken.

BAKED CHICKEN IN TOMATO BASIL SAUCE

1 4-pound chicken, cut into serving pieces
Lemon juice, salt, and pepper

Brush chicken with lemon juice and season with salt and pepper. Brown chicken well in a nonstick skillet and transfer pieces to a shallow baking dish. Pour Tomato Basil Sauce over the chicken.

Tomato Basil Sauce

Combine the following ingredients:

1 2-pound, 3-ounce can whole tomatoes,
  well-drained
2 large cloves garlic, minced
$1/2$ teaspoon thyme
$1/4$ cup chopped, fresh basil, or 1 teaspoon dried
$1/4$ cup red wine
$1/2$ teaspoon salt
$1/2$ teaspoon white pepper

Preheat oven to 350 degrees. Bake chicken and tomato sauce, covered, for 45 minutes and uncovered for 30 minutes. May be frozen or refrigerated. When ready to serve, bring to room temperature and bake at 350 degrees until heated through.

VEAL SCALLOPS MARINARA

8 ounces veal scallops
1 tablespoon olive oil
Salt and pepper

Dry veal thoroughly. Pour olive oil into a nonstick skillet. Add 2 veal scallops. Make sure scallops are not touching. (If they are crowded in the pan they will steam rather than fry to a nice brown.) Sauté for a few minutes on each side. Remove to a heated platter and keep warm while you prepare the other veal scallops. Season with salt and pepper. Serve with the following marinara sauce.

MARINARA SAUCE

This is a wonderful sauce and very easy to make. Use what you need for the veal and freeze the rest. It is equally good over fish or chicken.

1 onion, minced
1 tablespoon olive oil
1 clove garlic, minced
1 32-ounce can Italian plum tomatoes, drained and
    ground in food mill, or 1 can crushed tomatoes
1/2 teaspoon oregano
1 1/2 teaspoons basil
Salt and pepper
Drop of Tabasco sauce

In a nonstick saucepan, sauté the onion in margarine or vegetable oil until slightly browned. Add garlic, tomatoes, and herbs. Simmer, uncovered, for 30 minutes. Taste for seasoning.

VEAL WITH PAPRIKA AND PIMIENTO

1 pound ground veal
Salt and pepper
1 teaspoon dill
Imported paprika
Pimiento strips

Preheat broiler. Season veal with salt, pepper, and dill.
Shape veal into 4 patties and broil them until done on
each side. Sprinkle each with paprika and garnish with
pimiento strips. Serve hot. (This is also delicious prepared on a barbecue grill).

HONEY BARBECUE TEMPEH

*Serve this hearty dish over brown rice. For a low-fat
version, sauté the onions and garlic in water or vegetable
broth instead of oil.*

2 tablespoons olive oil
1 medium onion, coarsely chopped
3 cloves garlic, minced
1 14-ounce can unsalted tomatoes, drained and
    coarsely chopped, or chunky tomato sauce
2 tablespoons honey
1 tablespoon apple cider vinegar
2 tablespoons teriyaki sauce
1 teaspoon paprika
1 teaspoon ground cumin
8 ounces tempeh, steamed for 20 minutes and cut in
    1-inch strips, 1/4-inch thick

In a medium saucepan, sauté onion and garlic in
olive oil for 5 minutes. Add remaining ingredients and
simmer, partially covered, for 10 to 15 minutes or until
sauce thickens.

Red Vegetables

TOMATO CAULIFLOWER CASSEROLE

2 large heads cauliflower
2 tablespoons lemon juice
1 onion, minced
1 clove garlic, minced
1 16-ounce can Italian plum tomatoes, chopped
1 teaspoon salt
1/4 teaspoon pepper
1 teaspoon dried basil

Preheat oven to 350 degrees. Break cauliflowers into florets. Toss with lemon juice. Sauté onion and garlic in a nonstick pan until translucent. Add tomatoes, salt, pepper, and basil and heat through. Put cauliflower in a casserole dish and pour tomato mixture over. Bake uncovered for 40 minutes. Good hot or cold.

RED ITALIAN TOMATO CASSEROLE

This delicious salad is a perfect luncheon dish and can be made 1 hour in advance. Top with cottage cheese or minced hard-boiled eggs for a total meal.

4 large beefsteak tomatoes, sliced $1/2$-inch thick
1 red onion, sliced very thinly
Salt and freshly ground pepper
3 garlic cloves, minced
$1/4$ cup minced parsley
2 teaspoons fresh basil, or 1 teaspoon dried
2 tablespoons olive oil
2 tablespoon red wine vinegar

In a 3-quart casserole place a layer of tomato slices. Cover with onion slices. Sprinkle with salt and pepper and some of the garlic, parsley, and basil, a little of the oil and vinegar. Continue layering ingredients in this fashion until all are used. Refrigerate until well-chilled.

HERB BAKED TOMATOES

4 large tomatoes, halved
1 teaspoon fresh dill, or $1/2$ teaspoon dried
2 tablespoons minced, fresh parsley
1 teaspoon basil, dried
Salt and pepper

Preheat oven to 350 degrees. Place tomato halves in baking dish. Sprinkle each with herbs, salt, and pepper to taste. Bake for 10 minutes. Serve hot.

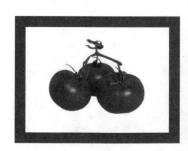

beauty

RED DAY BEAUTY TREATMENT

Cranberries and Rose Petals

Two beneficial, natural skin care ingredients on Red Day are cranberries and rose petals. Cranberry enzymes exfoliate dead skin cells so a healthier layer of skin can emerge. They also stimulate and refresh the skin, enhancing its natural tone.

Cranberry enzymes are beneficial for all skin types. For normal skin, the exfoliating cranberry enzymes maintain the natural balance of the skin, keeping the complexion bright. For dry skin, the enzymes digest dead skin cells that are just sitting on the surface. For oily skin, they unclog pores, absorbing excess oil for a clearer complexion. Pure Enzyme Mask by Cosmedix is good for all skin types and is an excellent exfoliate. Use it once a week.

Rose petals are both fragrant and soothing to the skin. Immerse fresh rose petals in warm water and then pour the water into a clean plastic spray bottle. After refrigerating for about three hours, mist your face and neck with the fresh rose water. This is particularly refreshing to the skin after a shower or after a workout. It will cool and calm your skin.

From the excitement of Red, think of all the lush greens of nature on Green Day. Bask in its tranquility and promise of a new you as you head into Day Three.

day 3 green

Green Day Sample Menu

Breakfast

Honeydew

Vanilla Milk Shake*

Coffee or tea

Lunch

Spinach Mushroom Salad with Yogurt Dill Dressing*

4 ounces dry tuna

Whole wheat bread, 1 slice

Herb tea

Snack

Granny Smith apple with 1 tablespoon peanut butter

Dinner

French Chicken in White Wine, 4 ounces*

Green Bean-Sprout Casserole, 1/2 cup*

Hot Spiced Pear, 1*

Decaffeinated coffee

Green Foods List

Green Fruits:
1 pear; honeydew, 1 cup frozen (unsweetened honeydew balls can be used); 1/4 cup green grapes; 1 small green apple

Green Vegetables:
Unlimited amounts of asparagus, broccoli, Brussels sprouts, cucumber, celery, chard, green beans, lettuce, spinach, zucchini

GREEN DAY RECIPES

Green Salads and Luncheon Dishes

GREEN DAY SALAD DRESSING

The following dressing is superb poured over a large, tossed green salad. Limit this to two tablespoons daily.

5 tablespoons dill, parsley, tarragon,
   and chives, mixed
¾ cup low-fat mayonnaise
¾ cup yogurt
2 tablespoons capers
Salt and pepper to taste

Put all ingredients in food processor or blender and blend until smooth. Pour over salad before serving. This makes 1½ cups of dressing. Can be stored in jar in the refrigerator for several days.

GREEN DAY CUCUMBER SALAD

Delicious as a side dish to cottage cheese, tuna, or a plain omelet.

1 medium cucumber, peeled, seeded, sliced
2 tablespoons wine vinegar
1 teaspoon salt
½ cup plain low-fat yogurt
1 tablespoon chopped, fresh dill
1 green onion

Toss cucumbers with salt and vinegar. Refrigerate one hour, stirring occasionally. Drain cucumbers well. Stir in yogurt, dill, and green onion. Toss to coat well and serve.

ORIENTAL CUCUMBER SALAD

Delicious salad as a side dish to baked fish. Unusual taste.

2 cucumbers, peeled, halved lengthwise, seeded
2 scallions, minced
1 tablespoon vinegar
1 teaspoon Splenda (artificial sweetener)
1 teaspoon soy sauce
1 teaspoon sesame oil
1/2 teaspoon salt
5 drops Tabasco sauce

Slice cucumbers thinly. Combine scallions, vinegar, sweetener, soy sauce, sesame oil, salt, and Tabasco sauce. Toss with cucumbers. Refrigerate. When ready to serve, place mound of cucumbers on bed of lettuce, sprinkling remaining sauce over lettuce.

CAULIFLOWER ONION SALAD WITH FRENCH DRESSING

1 cup thinly sliced raw cauliflower
1/2 cup thinly sliced onion
1/4 cup chopped green pepper
4 lettuce leaves, torn into bite-sized pieces
French dressing
Chopped scallions

French Dressing
Combine following ingredients
   in blender or food processor:

4 tablespoons wine vinegar
2 tablespoons salad oil
1 clove garlic, mashed
1/2 teaspoon salt
1/4 teaspoon pepper
1 teaspoon Dijon mustard

Toss together cauliflower, onion, green pepper, and lettuce. Moisten lightly with dressing. Sprinkle chopped scallions over salad.

SPINACH MUSHROOM SALAD WITH YOGURT DILL DRESSING

4 cups fresh spinach leaves, torn into pieces
2 cups fresh, sliced mushrooms
2 scallions, minced
4 hard-boiled eggs, chopped,
   or 6 cooked egg whites, chopped
Yogurt Dill Dressing

Yogurt Dill Dressing

Combine following ingredients
   in blender or food processor:

1 cup plain low-fat yogurt
2 tablespoons fresh dill
1 clove garlic
1/2 teaspoon Dijon mustard
Salt and pepper to taste

In a large salad bowl toss spinach, mushrooms, scallions, and chopped eggs. Top with Yogurt Dill Dressing before serving and toss well.

CHEESE SPINACH PIE

1 10-ounce package frozen chopped spinach,
   cooked and drained well
1 cup cottage cheese
2 eggs, beaten, or 4 egg whites, beaten
1 teaspoon seasoned salt
1/4 teaspoon seasoned pepper
1/4 teaspoon nutmeg

Preheat oven to 350 degrees. Mix all ingredients together. Place in very lightly greased, 8-inch pie pan. Sprinkle with paprika. Bake for 30 minutes or until set.

MUSHROOM AND ZUCCHINI SALAD

2 cups thinly sliced zucchini
1/2 pound fresh mushrooms, thinly sliced
2 tablespoons fresh lemon juice
2 tablespoons minced parsley
1 clove garlic, mashed
1/2 cup plain low-fat yogurt
1 teaspoon Dijon mustard
1 teaspoon salt
1/2 teaspoon freshly ground black pepper

Toss zucchini and mushrooms with lemon juice and minced parsley to coat evenly. In blender combine garlic, yogurt, Dijon mustard, salt, and pepper. Pour over vegetables right before serving.

INDIAN COLESLAW

4 cups thinly shredded cabbage
1/2 cup diced celery
1/2 cup diced green pepper
1/2 cup minced scallions
3 tablespoons minced, fresh parsley
2 tablespoons wine vinegar
2 tablespoons fresh lemon juice
1 tablespoon Dijon mustard
1 teaspoon salt
1 teaspoon sugar, or 1 packet artificial sweetener
2 bay leaves, pulverized
1/2 teaspoon cumin seed
1/4 cup low-fat mayonnaise
1/2 cup low-fat yogurt

Toss together cabbage, celery, green pepper, scallions, and parsley. In blender puree vinegar, lemon juice, mustard, salt, sugar or sweetener, bay leaves, cumin seed, mayonnaise, and yogurt. Pour dressing over cabbage, toss well, and chill.

MIDDLE EASTERN COLESLAW

Delicious made in advance and allowed to marinate.

1 small green cabbage, shredded
1 small green pepper, thinly sliced
1 small onion, thinly sliced
3 tablespoons chopped parsley
3 tablespoons chopped, fresh mint
1/4 cup lemon juice
2 tablespoons olive oil
1 large clove garlic, mashed
1/2 teaspoon white pepper
1 teaspoon salt

Combine cabbage, green pepper, onion, parsley, and mint in large salad bowl. Beat together lemon juice, oil, garlic, pepper, and salt until well blended. Pour dressing over vegetables and toss gently.

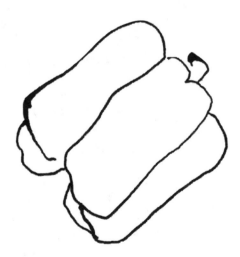

GREEN DAY VEGETABLE SALAD WITH DRESSING

This dressing is delicious poured over a variety of vegetables that are either lightly steamed or served raw. My favorite combination is to toss together cauliflower, string beans, and broccoli that I have lightly steamed. I serve this as a luncheon salad with the dressing poured over it right before serving.

1 head cauliflower, broken into florets
1 pound string beans, broken into 2-inch pieces
1 pound broccoli, broken into florets

Dressing

12 ounces regular cottage cheese
1/2 small onion
2 cucumbers, peeled and seeded
2 teaspoons dill
1 clove garlic
3 tablespoons wine vinegar
1 tablespoon Vegit seasoning

Puree all dressing ingredients in blender or food processor until creamy.

Green Soups

ZUCCHINI SOUP

This soup is delicious served either hot or cold. It is just as good made with cucumbers or asparagus.

$1/2$ onion, chopped
1 tablespoon margarine
2 cups zucchini, cut into chunks
3 cups chicken broth
1 teaspoon farina (optional)
1 teaspoon white wine vinegar
1 teaspoon fresh tarragon (or $1/2$ teaspoon dried)
Salt and pepper to taste

In a large saucepan, sauté onion in margarine until tender and transparent. Add zucchini, chicken broth, farina, wine vinegar, and tarragon. Season with salt and pepper. Simmer covered for 30 minutes. Puree this mixture in blender or food processor.

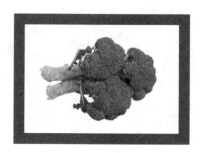

CUCUMBER AND STRING BEAN SOUP

This is a delightful cold soup. It is a perfect prelude to a light lunch or dinner.

1/4 pound string beans
1 large cucumber, cut into chunks
1 large clove garlic
2 cups plain low-fat yogurt
Salt and white pepper to taste
Dill, dried or fresh, to garnish

Blanch string beans in boiling, salted water for 5 to 7 minutes or until tender. Drain and run under cold water to stop the cooking process. Place string beans, cucumber, and garlic in a blender or food processor and blend until smooth. Add the yogurt to cucumber mixture and blend well. Refrigerate until well chilled. At serving time, season with salt, white pepper, and dill.

CUCUMBER BISQUE

1 tablespoon olive oil
1/2 cup finely chopped onion
1 tablespoon flour
3 large cucumbers, peeled and chopped
3 cups vegetable stock
1 cup yogurt
2 small cucumbers, peeled and diced
Salt and pepper to taste
1/4 cup finely chopped parsley

In a 2 1/2-quart saucepan, heat olive oil and sauté onion without browning. Stir in flour and add chopped cucumbers. Blend well and when hot add vegetable stock. Bring to a boil, cover, and simmer over low heat about 45 minutes. Cool slightly, and puree in blender. Let chill. When cold, stir in yogurt with a wire whisk. Add remaining cucumber, salt and pepper to taste, and parsley. Serve soup well chilled.

Green Protein Dishes

SPANISH BAKED FISH

2 pounds fish fillets (sea bass, sole, haddock,
   or flounder)
1 large clove garlic, minced
1 green pepper, minced
1 onion, sliced in rings
1 tablespoon olive oil
1 tablespoon white wine vinegar
1 teaspoon dried oregano
Paprika
Salt and pepper

Preheat oven to 350 degrees. Lay fish fillets in a nonstick baking dish. Sprinkle with garlic, green pepper,
and onion rings. Mix oil, vinegar, and oregano and
pour over all. Sprinkle with paprika, salt, and pepper.
Bake, covered, for 30 minutes.

HERB BAKED FISH

2 pounds fish fillets
Juice of 1 lemon
1 tablespoon butter or margarine
1 teaspoon white pepper
1 teaspoon Vegit seasoning (or seasoned salt)
1 cup white wine
1 tablespoon minced, fresh parsley
1 tablespoon minced, fresh dill
1 tablespoon minced, fresh basil

Preheat oven to 350 degrees. Roll fish in lemon juice
and place in lightly buttered baking dish. Season fish
with pepper and salt. Pour wine over fish and sprinkle
with herbs. Bake covered for 30 minutes.

GREEN DAY ROAST CHICKEN

This recipe was given to me by my friend Vera Loeffler, who is one of the finest cooks I know.

1 large green pepper
1 large onion
2 stalks celery
1 3-pound chicken, cut into serving pieces
1 tablespoon paprika
1 teaspoon salt
1 teaspoon white pepper
1 teaspoon thyme

Preheat oven to 375 degrees. Slice green pepper, onion, and celery into thick strips. Make a bed of these vegetables in a shallow casserole. Season chicken well with paprika, salt, pepper, and thyme. Place on a bed of vegetables. Bake for 45 minutes, uncovered. Cover and bake 30 minutes longer.

FRENCH CHICKEN IN WHITE WINE

This chicken dish is easy, delicious, and a very special one to share with friends.

1 4-pound chicken, cut into serving pieces
1 tablespoon oil
1 onion, chopped
1 green pepper, chopped
2 celery stalks, thinly sliced
2 tablespoons fresh dill, or 1 tablespoon dried
1 teaspoon savory
1 teaspoon white pepper
1 tablespoon paprika
1 tablespoon Vegit seasoning (or seasoned salt)
1/2 cup chicken broth
1 cup dry white wine

Preheat oven to 350 degrees. In nonstick casserole brown chicken well. When well browned remove to another platter. In the same skillet sauté onion, green pepper, and celery. Season chicken with dill, savory, white pepper, paprika, and Vegit salt and return to skillet. Pour broth and wine over the chicken. Cover. Bake in oven for 1 1/2 hours.

Green Vegetables

GREEN DAY STEAMED VEGETABLES

Vegetables on Green Day are delicious eaten hot or cold. The simplest way to prepare them is to simply place them on a vegetable steamer in a pot with a lid. Add 1 to 2 cups water to the pot and bring to a boil. Turn water off and let vegetables steam for 10 to 15 minutes. They should be crunchy and beautiful to look at, as this method helps them retain their gorgeous color.

The vegetables are perfect unadorned, but, if you wish, you may sprinkle lightly with some lemon juice, fresh herbs, salt, and pepper to taste.

Vegetables

Enjoy the vegetables that are in season: asparagus in spring, green beans in summer, broccoli all year long. Lightly steamed vegetables are filling, tasty, and pretty.

BROCCOLI GREEN BEAN CASSEROLE

3 cups water
1 pound broccoli, broken into florets, leaves removed
1 pound green beans, ends snapped
   and broken into pieces
Juice of 1 lemon
1/4 cup chopped, fresh herbs (parsley, dill, basil)
Salt and pepper to taste

In large pot, put vegetable steamer and 3 cups water. Place vegetables on steaming rack, cover pot, and bring water to a boil. When water boils, turn off heat and let vegetables steam for 10 to 15 minutes. Drain vegetables and season with lemon juice, herbs, salt, and pepper. Good hot or cold.

GREEN BEAN CRUNCH

Excellent cold vegetable dish that can be made well in advance to accompany fish or chicken.

1 1/2 cups water
1/2 teaspoon salt
1 small onion, cut into quarters
1 large clove garlic
2 1/2 pounds green beans, washed
   and cut into 2-inch pieces
1/2 cup soy sauce
1 tablespoon safflower oil

Bring water to a boil in a heavy, covered saucepan with salt, onion, and garlic. Add green beans; return to boil. Cover and cook over low heat 5 minutes. Drain well and remove garlic.

Blend together soy sauce and 1 tablespoon oil and add to beans, tossing gently. Let beans marinate 1 hour in refrigerator. Toss again before serving.

GREEN BEAN-SPROUT CASSEROLE

1 pound fresh green beans
3 cups bean sprouts
2 tablespoon wine vinegar
1 teaspoon Dijon mustard
1 clove garlic, crushed
3 tablespoons olive oil
3 tablespoons minced herbs (parsley, tarragon, dill)
Salt and pepper to taste

Snap ends of beans, wash, and steam for 10 minutes until crunchy. Rinse under cold water to refresh them and stop the cooking. In colander wash bean sprouts. Pour boiling water over them to soften. Combine sprouts with green beans. In glass jar combine vinegar, mustard, garlic, oil, and minced herbs. Pour over green beans and sprouts. Season well with salt and freshly ground pepper. Refrigerate and let marinate until ready to serve.

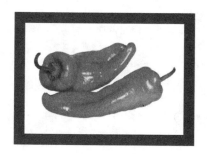

beauty

Cucumbers, Green Tea, and Olive Oil

One of the best soothers for skin is cucumber, which can be used straight from the refrigerator and is beneficial for all skin types. Cut into slices, cold cucumbers soothe tired eyes and cool aggravated, reddened skin. Great for use during a bath or before bed, cucumber slices have an anti-inflammatory effect on the skin. After a long day of work or a difficult "cry-fest," there is nothing better than lying down with cold cucumber slices over your eyes and face to calm *everything* down.

Another way to relax with some natural green products is to make use of the green tea bags you have in your kitchen cabinet. Green tea, an antioxidant, is an excellent ingredient to soothe skin irritated by environmental factors, such as sun exposure. Soak the green tea bags in warm water, remove the excess water, let cool and place on eyes and face for up to ten minutes. Your skin will feel younger and healthier immediately.

Another easy way to relax the natural way is to rub olive oil into your feet, put on a pair of white cotton socks, and leave them on overnight. The olive oil will infuse your skin, hydrating the surface of your feet and soothing your soles. After a long day, your feet deserve only the best!

Now step into sensuous Orange Day, a color so vibrant and rich, it can satisfy your appetite. Revel in the orange foods on this Day Four of your 7-Day Color Diet, but keep your portions under control.

day 4 orange

Orange Day Sample Menu

Breakfast

Peach Milk Shake*

Add a Beige

Coffee or tea

Lunch

Orange Day Coleslaw, 1 cup*

Omelet, 2 whole eggs

Whole wheat toast, 1 slice

5 dried apricots

Herb tea

Snack

1 ounce low-fat cheddar cheese
  on a slice of whole wheat toast

Dinner

Spanish Orange Fish Fillets, 4 ounces*

Marinated Carrot Casserole, $1/2$ cup*

Oranges in Red Wine, 1 cup,*
  or 4 ounces orange sorbet

Decaffeinated coffee

Orange Foods List

Orange Fruits:
1 orange or $1/2$ cup
orange juice;
$1/2$ cantaloupe;
1 mango; 1 fresh
peach or $1/2$ cup
canned in its own
juice; $1/2$ papaya;
2 fresh apricots or
4 halves canned
in their own juice;
1 tangerine;
1 nectarine

Orange Vegetables:
Unlimited amounts
of carrots

ORANGE DAY RECIPES

Orange Salads and Luncheon Dishes

ORANGE DAY CARROT SALAD

1 cup cottage cheese
2 large carrots, shredded
1 orange, cut into bite-sized pieces
1 teaspoon cinnamon
1/3 cup yogurt
4 tablespoons orange juice
1 tablespoon freshly grated orange peel

Mix cottage cheese with carrots, orange pieces, and cinnamon. Mix yogurt with orange juice and orange peel. Serve as a dressing on the side to cottage cheese mixture.

ORANGE DAY COLESLAW

Inspired by Minnie Miller—better known as "Aunt Minnie."

2 large carrots, shredded
1 large white cabbage, shredded
1/4 cup mayonnaise
1/4 cup yogurt
2 tablespoons wine vinegar
1 teaspoon celery seed
1 teaspoon seasoned salt
1/2 teaspoon pepper
1 packet artificial sweetener or 1 teaspoon sugar

Put shredded carrots and cabbage in a large bowl. Mix mayonnaise, yogurt, wine vinegar, celery seed, salt and pepper, and sweetener. Pour over coleslaw. Serve well chilled.

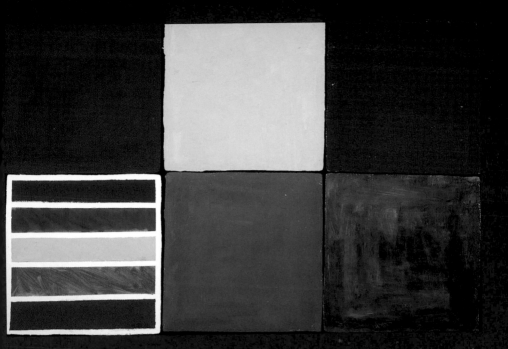

Like seven days at a lovely health spa–The 7-Day Color Diet offers you a healthy color-a-day diet plan that will help you reach your weight loss goals, one color at a time. From White through Red, Green, Orange, Purple, and Yellow and into Rainbow Day, savor the rich spectrum of nature's colors as you lose unwanted pounds and gain the healthiest of complexions. By the end of the first week, you'll be slimmer, more energetic, and glowing with health. The Color Diet is easy, fun, and colorful; it tastes good, looks good, and is good for you—what more can you ask? Besides that, it works!

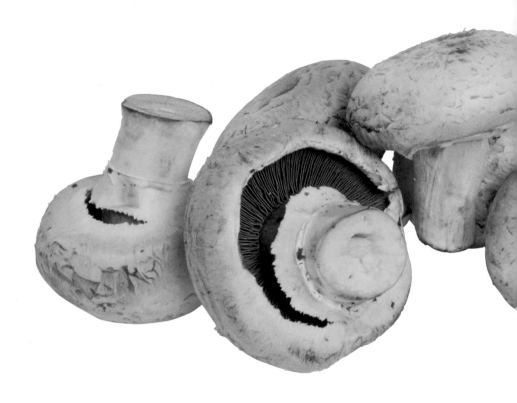

day 1/white

This is Day 1 of your colorful new way of eating. Today you'll eat only white foods like white grapefruit, mushrooms, onions in dishes like Roast Chicken with Herbs. After White Day, you'll be adding glorious color after color, as you lose pound after pound. On this day, start with a Vanilla Honey Milk Shake and end with a cleansing and hydrating skin treatment.

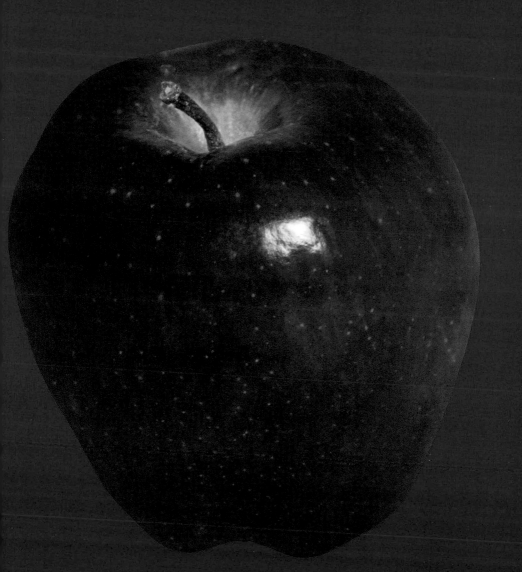

day 2/red

On Day 2, you will move into the most exciting of all colors—red. Relish the flavors of these sensual red foods such as strawberries, apples, raspberries, watermelon; Iced Tomato Soup and Red Day Sole Provencal. See all your recipe choices starting on page 49, then treat your skin to beauty with cranberries and rose petals.

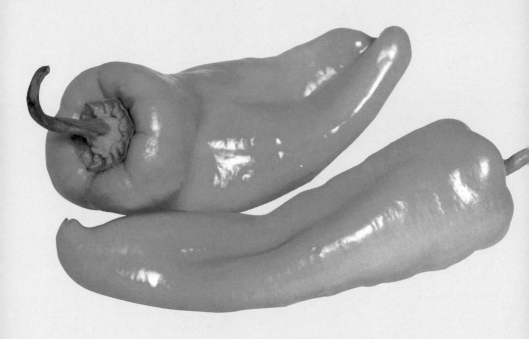

day 3/green

On Green Day 3, bask in the tranquility and promise of a new you. Bite into honeydew melon, green grapes, and pears; delight in Cheese Spinach Pie or Cucumber Green Bean Soup. Soothe your tired skin with cucumber slices and green tea. You'll find much that is delicious and green, on page 65.

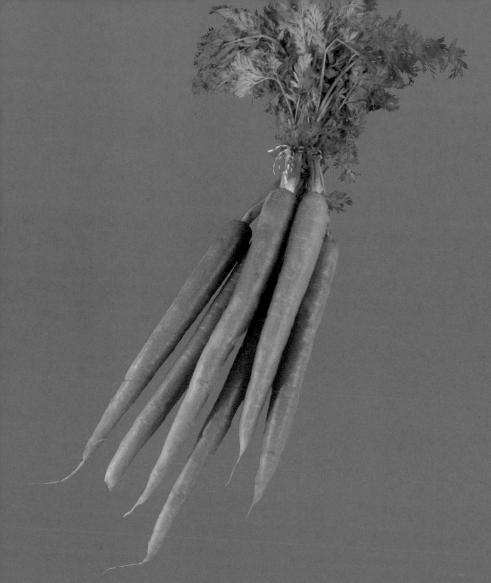

day 4/orange

On Day 4, step into sensuous Orange. Revel in such orange fruits as canteloupes, peaches, and tangerines; try Spanish Orange Fish Fillets and Curried Carrot Soup or Carrot Kugelhopf on this Day 4 of your Color Diet. The fun and the recipes begin on page 81.

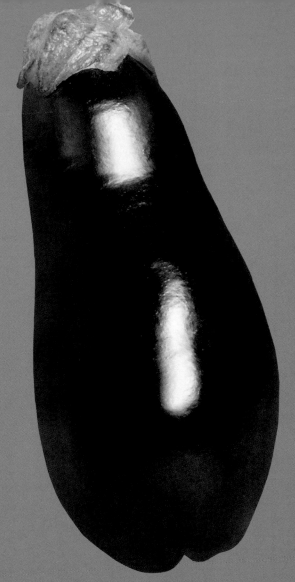

day 5/purple

Let the cool, romantic color of purple work its magic on Day 5. From plums, blueberries, and blackberries to Chicken in Plum Sauce and Purple Cabbage Slaw, this is a day rich in color. Soothe your face with lovely lavender essence. Purple Day begins on page 105.

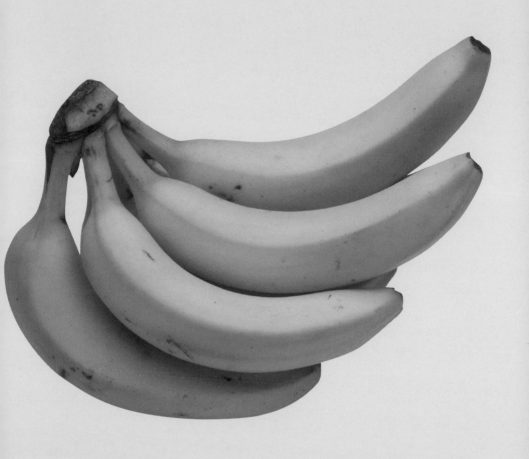

day 6/yellow

On Yellow Day 6, be happy with everything from your morning Pineapple Milk Shake, to Roast Chicken with Mustard and Herbs, and Yellow Squash Soup. Tighten, lighten, and brighten your skin with a Vitamin C serum. Yellow's delights begin on page 119.

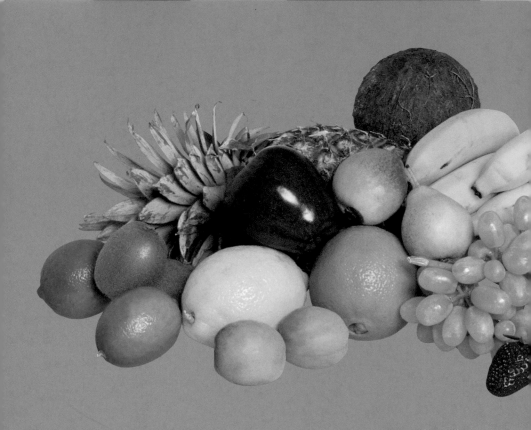

day 7/rainbow

This is the celebrate-all-colors day—the end of your first week on the 7-Day Color Diet. After Rainbow Day, you may repeat all the colors of the first week, then move on to the maintenance plan if you have met your weight loss goal. Of course, the Rainbow Food List consists of all the foods from the other six Color Days, but now you may dig into Rainbow Salad Nicoise and Rainbow Stir-fry Vegetables. Treat yourself to an oatmeal bath or clay mask. Already you are glowing!

Orange Soups

CURRIED CARROT SOUP

1 pound carrots, cut into chunks
1 small onion, minced
2 cups chicken broth
1 cup water from steamed carrots
1 teaspoon white wine vinegar
1 teaspoon imported curry powder
$1/4$ teaspoon cumin
Pinch of cinnamon

Steam the carrots until tender, and save the water. Using a nonstick pan or nonstick spray, sauté the onion until tender.

Add carrots, chicken broth, carrot water, vinegar, curry, cumin, and cinnamon, and simmer for 15 minutes. Puree in a blender, food processor, or food mill. Test for seasoning. Serve hot.

COLD ORANGE-CARROT SOUP

1/2 cup minced onion
1 strip orange peel
1 tablespoon butter
2 teaspoons flour
2 cups sliced carrots
2 1/2 cups water
1 teaspoon sugar
1/2 teaspoon salt
1/4 teaspoon ground ginger
1/4 teaspoon ground cloves
1 1/2 cups orange juice
1 tablespoon lemon juice
White pepper to taste
1/4 cup plain low-fat yogurt
Finely chopped mint or chives

Cook onion and orange peel slowly in butter until soft. Stir in flour until smooth. Add carrots, water, sugar, salt, and spices. Cover and cook gently until tender enough to puree (about 10 minutes). Puree in blender until smooth. Add orange juice, lemon juice, white pepper, and yogurt. Blend until smooth. Cover and chill. Serve cold with chopped mint or chives sprinkled on top.

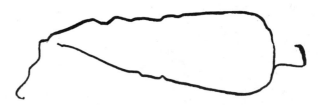

COLD CARROT SOUP

1 pound carrots, thinly sliced
1 leek, white part only, sliced
1/2 teaspoon grated, fresh ginger
1 tablespoon oil
3 cups chicken broth
1/2 teaspoon salt
3/4 cup orange juice

Sauté carrots, leek, and ginger in oil until soft. Add chicken broth and salt, cover, and simmer for about 30 minutes. Puree in blender or processor. Add orange juice and chill. Stir before serving.

Orange Protein Dishes

FISH AND CARROT BAKE

2 pounds fillet of sole
Salt, pepper, and paprika
2 large scallions, minced
1 garlic clove, minced
1 cup sliced carrots
1/4 cup chopped, fresh parsley
1/2 cup dry white wine

Preheat oven to 350 degrees. In nonstick casserole lay fish fillets flat. Season well with salt, pepper, and paprika. Top with scallions, garlic, carrots, and parsley. Pour wine over all and bake, covered, for 30 minutes.

SPANISH ORANGE FISH FILLETS

2 large oranges, peeled
3 pounds bass fillets
2 tablespoons butter
Salt and white pepper
1 tablespoon minced onion
$1/2$ cup orange juice
$1/2$ cup dry white wine
1 teaspoon grated orange rind

Segment the two oranges and set aside. Sauté fish in
butter until fish flakes easily. Sprinkle with salt and
pepper to taste and keep warm on separate platter.
Cook onion in butter remaining in pan until soft. Stir
in orange juice, wine, and grated rind. Season with salt
and pepper and simmer for 5 minutes. Add orange
segments and heat through. Arrange orange segments
around the fillets on platter and pour sauce over fish.
Serve hot.

ORANGE DAY ESCABECHE

An easy, tasty luncheon dish to prepare a day in advance. It improves in flavor as it marinates. This looks lovely served on crisp lettuce greens and garnished with lemon and orange slices.

2 pounds flounder fillets
1 tablespoon lemon juice
1 clove garlic, crushed
3 tablespoons lemon juice, freshly squeezed
3/4 cup orange juice
1/4 cup minced scallions
1/2 teaspoon ground cumin seed
Dash of Tabasco sauce
1 tablespoon olive oil
Salt and freshly ground white pepper to taste

Dip the fish in lemon juice and sauté in nonstick skillet, covered, for 8 to 10 minutes on each side. Remove to glass dish. In saucepan, combine garlic, lemon juice, orange juice, scallions, cumin seed, Tabasco sauce, olive oil, salt, and pepper. Pour over fish and let stand in refrigerator for 24 hours.

ORANGE DAY SALMON MOUSSE

Good luncheon dish.

1 envelope unflavored gelatin
1 1/4 cups water
1 15 1/2-ounce can salmon, drained and flaked
3/4 cup chopped celery
1/3 cup low-fat mayonnaise
1/2 cup chopped parsley
2 tablespoons lemon juice
1 teaspoon grated lemon peel
1 teaspoon grated onion
1 teaspoon celery seed

Sprinkle gelatin over water; heat and stir until dissolved. Remove from heat and refrigerate until slightly thickened. When gelatin is ready, combine with salmon, celery, mayonnaise, parsley, lemon juice and peel, onion, and celery seed. Pour into glass bowl. Serve well chilled.

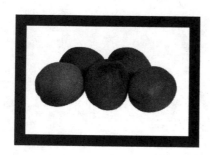

PERSIAN CHICKEN WITH PEACHES

This is excellent!

2 chickens, cut into quarters
2 teaspoons salt
2 teaspoons rosemary
1 can (29 ounces) cling peaches, packed in their own
    juice. (Reserve juice.)
1 tablespoon honey
2 tablespoons minced onion
1 teaspoon curry powder
1 teaspoon powdered ginger (optional)

Preheat oven to 425 degrees. Pat chicken dry. Sprinkle
with salt and rosemary. In nonstick baking pan, bake
chicken skin side down for 45 minutes. While chicken
is baking, prepare glaze. In saucepan, combine peaches
and juice, honey, onion, curry, and ginger. Simmer
5 minutes. Turn chicken pieces over skin side up.
Cover heavily with glaze and bake 30 minutes more.
Baste with glaze once or twice. Serve hot.

ORANGE DAY CHICKEN CURRY

1 4-pound chicken, cut into serving pieces
1 teaspoon salt
1 teaspoon pepper
1 onion, chopped
4 carrots, thickly sliced
3/4 cup orange juice
3/4 cup chicken broth
1 bay leaf, crumbled
1 tablespoon curry powder
1 teaspoon celery salt
1 naval orange, sectioned

Season chicken with salt and pepper. In large nonstick skillet, brown chicken. Remove chicken pieces and keep warm. In the same skillet add onion, carrots, orange juice, chicken broth, bay leaf, curry, and celery salt. Return chicken pieces to skillet. Reduce heat and simmer, covered, one hour. Garnish with orange segments.

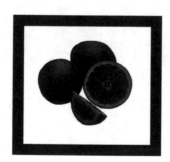

Orange Vegetables

ORANGE PUMPKIN PUDDING

1$\frac{1}{2}$ packages Mori-Nu Silken Lite Tofu Firm (for firmer
   texture use Mori-Nu Silken Lite Tofu Extra-Firm)
1$\frac{1}{2}$ cups canned or cooked pumpkin
$\frac{1}{4}$ cup honey
1 teaspoon vanilla extract
1 tablespoon Pumpkin Pie Spice, or next 4 ingredients
1$\frac{1}{2}$ teaspoons ground cinnamon
$\frac{3}{4}$ teaspoon ground ginger
$\frac{1}{4}$ teaspoon ground nutmeg
$\frac{1}{4}$ teaspoon ground cloves

Preheat oven to 400 degrees. Blend Mori-Nu Silken Lite
Tofu Firm in a food processor or blender until creamy
smooth. Add pumpkin, honey, vanilla, and spices; blend
well. Pour into a 9-inch Pyrex dish. Bake approximately
1 hour or until a toothpick inserted in the center comes
out almost clean. Can be served hot or cold.

MARINATED CARROT CASSEROLE

*The secret of this delicious marinated carrot dish is to
toss the carrots in the dressing and herbs while they are
still hot. The carrots absorb all the flavors of the dressing.
This is a beautiful dish for a buffet. It is superb.*

4 cups tiny carrots, peeled
2 cups water
1/2 teaspoon salt
1 tablespoon fresh tarragon or 1 teaspoon dried
1 tablespoon finely chopped parsley
2 tablespoons chopped scallions
1 clove garlic, crushed
4 tablespoons dry white wine
1 tablespoon oil
1 tablespoon lemon juice
Freshly ground black pepper

Put carrots in heavy saucepan with water and salt.
Cover and bring water to a boil. Reduce heat immediately and cook gently for 10 minutes. Carrots should be
tender but still crunchy. Drain and save liquid to make
soup for another day. Mix together tarragon, parsley,
scallions, garlic, wine, oil, and lemon juice. Cook for 5
minutes. Coat carrots lightly with this dressing. Season
with freshly ground pepper. Chill carrots well and serve
in a pretty glass bowl. This casserole can be served hot
as well.

ORANGE DAY CARROTS

8 medium carrots, cut into thick slices
1/2 teaspoon salt
1/2 cup boiling water
1/4 cup orange juice
1 teaspoon grated orange peel
1 tablespoon chopped scallion, white part only
1 orange, peeled and cut into bite-sized pieces

Cook carrots, covered, in boiling salted water until tender, but crunchy, 10 to 15 minutes. Drain. Toss carrots until well coated with juice, orange peel, scallion, and orange pieces. Serve hot or cold.

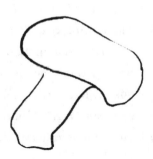

CARROT KUGELHOPF

This dish has all your vegetables and protein to serve as a one-dish meal. It is delicious for lunch or dinner.

1 tablespoon olive oil
2 cloves garlic, minced
4 scallions, chopped
8 carrots, thinly sliced
1 1/2 cups boiling vegetable stock
1/2 teaspoon turmeric
1/4 teaspoon salt
1/4 teaspoon pepper
4 or 6 egg whites
2 cups mushrooms, diced
1 cup grated low-fat Swiss cheese, firmly packed
2 tablespoons finely chopped parsley

Preheat oven to 375 degrees. In a large saucepan, heat olive oil. Sauté garlic and scallions. Add carrots and stock. Cover and simmer until carrots are soft, about 30 minutes. Remove cover and cook on low heat until liquid evaporates. Mash carrots coarsely and stir in turmeric, salt, pepper, and eggs until thoroughly blended. Add mushrooms, cheese, and parsley. Turn carrot and cheese mixture into a lightly oiled 6-cup casserole. Place casserole in a pan half filled with hot water and bake 45 minutes. Serve hot.

beauty

ORANGE DAY BEAUTY TREATMENT
Papayas

A great skin care ingredient is *papain*, a naturally

occurring enzyme in papayas. This enzyme, like that of

cranberries, exfoliates the complexion for all skin types.

Papain cleanses away dead skin cells and allows a

brighter, healthier layer of skin to emerge. Papain

enzyme is found in powder and liquid form products.

Dermalogica Daily Microfoliant can be used for all skin

types. Use it once a week as an exfoliate.

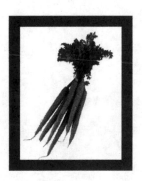

Though purple is a cool color, especially after your Orange Day, to many it is a royal and romantic color. Let it work its magic on you as you enter Day Five of the Color Diet.

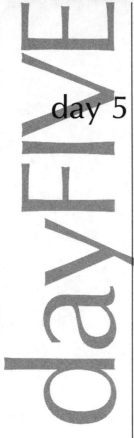

day 5 purple

Purple Day Sample Menu

Breakfast

Blueberry Milk Shake*

Add a Beige

Coffee or tea

Lunch

Purple Day Beet and Egg Salad, 1 cup*

Whole wheat toast, 1 slice

Herb tea

Snack

4 ounces raspberry yogurt with $1/2$ ounce raisins

Dinner

Cauliflower Beet Casserole, $1/2$ cup*

Chicken with Plum Sauce, 4 ounces*

Water chestnuts

4 ounces raspberry sorbet, topped
with a sprinkling of blueberries

Decaffeinated coffee

Purple Foods Lists

Purple Fruits:

2 fresh or canned
plums, juice pack;
1 cup blueberries;
1 cup blackberries

Purple Vegetables:

Unlimited amounts
of beets, eggplant,
purple cabbage

PURPLE DAY RECIPES

Purple Salads and Luncheon Dishes

PURPLE DAY BEET AND EGG SALAD

Excellent lunch!

1 cup shredded, cooked beets
3 hard-boiled eggs, chopped
2 tablespoons chopped onion
1 tablespoon fresh dill
2 tablespoons plain low-fat yogurt
1 tablespoon low-fat mayonnaise

Mix all ingredients together and mound
on bed of salad greens.

PURPLE CABBAGE SLAW

1 medium purple cabbage, shredded

Dressing
1/4 cup low-fat mayonnaise
1/4 cup plain low-fat yogurt
1/2 small onion, minced
1 tablespoon cider vinegar
1 teaspoon salt
1/4 teaspoon freshly ground pepper
1 teaspoon celery seed
1 packet Splenda (artificial sweetener),
    or 1 teaspoon sugar

Blend dressing ingredients. Pour over cabbage. Top with
cottage cheese for a delicious Purple Day lunch.

CHOPPED EGGPLANT SALAD

This eggplant salad is delicious served as a side to roast chicken or broiled fish. It is also tasty as a luncheon dish mixed with finely chopped hard-boiled eggs.

1 eggplant, unpeeled
$1/2$ teaspoon salt
$1/2$ teaspoon pepper
2 tablespoons lemon juice
2 tablespoons parsley
1 tablespoon oil
2 tablespoons chopped onion
1 garlic clove, minced

Preheat oven to 450 degrees. Bake eggplant whole and unpeeled for 30 to 40 minutes. Peel and chop eggplant. Add salt, pepper, lemon juice, parsley, oil, onion, and garlic. Stir well and chill.

Purple Soups

CHERRY SOY SOUP

Cherries are their best in the summer. You can eat them right off the stems, use them in pies, or as toppings for desserts. I designed this creamy cherry soup to add elegance to this popular summer fruit.

3 cans purple cherries, drained
1 teaspoon vanilla extract
1 cup water
2 teaspoons lemon juice
$\frac{1}{4}$ teaspoon cinnamon
2 cups plain soy milk

In a saucepan over medium high heat, simmer the cherries in the vanilla and water until they are soft, about 10 minutes. Stir occasionally. While the cherries are simmering, add lemon juice and cinnamon; mix thoroughly. Transfer the cherry mixture to a food processor or blender and puree until it forms a thick liquid. It also should be cooling down. When the mixture reaches room temperature, add soy milk and continue to puree. Serve chilled.

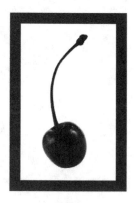

TOBEE'S BORSCHT

This soup is delicious as well as beautiful.

5 medium-sized beets, unpeeled
Water
1/2 cup lemon juice, fresh
1 teaspoon salt
Sugar substitute to taste
5 eggs, well beaten in large mixing bowl

Scrub beets well and put into a large soup pot. Cover with water. Bring to a boil. Reduce heat and simmer 45 minutes. Remove beets and discard water. Let beets cool so that skins can be easily slipped off. Grate beets into soup pot and cover with cold water. Bring to boil. When beets come to a rolling boil add lemon juice, salt, and sugar substitute to taste. (The soup should have a sweet-sour flavor—adjust with more lemon or sweetener according to your taste.) With a hand mixer, beat one cup of the borscht liquid into the beaten eggs. Keep adding more borscht and beat until the eggs and borscht are well blended. Refrigerate until ready to serve. Serve well chilled.

CHILLED BEET SOUP

1 cup low-fat yogurt
1 16-ounce can diced beets. (Reserve liquid.)
3 teaspoons vegetable bouillon granules dissolved in
   2 cups boiling water
1 tablespoon dark brown sugar
1 tablespoon lemon juice
$1/2$ teaspoon salt
$1/8$ teaspoon white pepper
2 small scallions, thinly sliced
Several sprigs fresh dill, minced

Pour yogurt into a medium bowl. Whisk together
yogurt, beet liquid, bouillon stock, sugar, lemon juice,
salt, pepper, and scallions. Add diced beets. Chill soup
well and garnish with minced dill.

Purple Fish Dishes

TUNA STUFFED EGGPLANT

1 medium eggplant
Salt
1 tablespoon olive oil or mayonnaise
$1/4$ cup fresh bread crumbs
2 tablespoons minced, fresh parsley
2 garlic cloves, mashed
1 cup tuna, well drained and finely minced
1 teaspoon dried oregano
Salt to taste
Freshly ground black pepper
1 tablespoon well-drained capers

Preheat oven to 350 degrees. Rinse the eggplants and
cut them in half lengthwise. Make 3 large slits in each
half. Sprinkle with salt and put on paper towels to
drain. Let drain for 1 hour. Dry thoroughly and place
on baking sheet. Bake in oven for 30 minutes or until

tender. Remove eggplant. When cool enough to handle, scoop out the flesh without breaking the skin. Place shells in a nonstick casserole and set aside. Finely mince the eggplant pulp. Combine eggplant in a mixing bowl with bread crumbs, parsley, garlic, tuna, and oregano. Blend thoroughly with a fork. Season with salt and pepper. Fill eggplant shells with the tuna mixture. Bake for 20 minutes. Remove the dish and cool completely. Garnish with capers.

Purple Chicken Dishes

CHICKEN WITH PLUM SAUCE AND WATER CHESTNUTS

1 2½-pound fryer cut into serving pieces
Salt
Pepper
1 16-ounce can unsweetened
   purple plums. (Reserve liquid.)
1 cup chicken stock
1 clove garlic, minced
2 tablespoons soy sauce
2 tablespoons cider vinegar
½ cup water chestnuts, sliced

Preheat oven to 350 degrees. Season chicken with salt and pepper. Brown on top of the stove in a nonstick casserole. Arrange chicken pieces side by side in casserole. Combine plums, 1 cup plum liquid, chicken stock, garlic, soy sauce, cider vinegar, and water chestnuts. Pour over chicken. Bake covered for 1 hour or until chicken is tender.

CHICKEN WITH EGGPLANT

1 2- to 3-pound chicken, cut up into serving pieces
Salt
Pepper
1 tablespoon olive oil
1 large eggplant, peeled and cubed
1/4 pound mushrooms, sliced
1 large onion, chopped
2 cloves garlic, minced
1/4 teaspoon basil
1/4 teaspoon thyme
1/2 teaspoon salt
1 1/2 cups chicken broth
1/2 cup red wine

Preheat oven to 350 degrees. Season chicken with salt
and pepper. In nonstick skillet, brown chicken well in
oil and set aside. Add eggplant, mushrooms, onion, and
garlic to skillet. Put chicken pieces on top and sprinkle
with basil, thyme, and salt. Pour broth and wine over
all. Cover and bake 1 1/2 hours.

Purple Vegetables

SOYBEAN VEGETARIAN MOUSSAKA

This recipe began with an idea for vegetarian Moussaka and evolved into a simple and colorful summer casserole that's good warm or at room temperature. You can substitute garbanzo beans for the soybeans.

1 onion, chopped
2 cloves garlic, minced
1 tablespoon olive oil
1 medium eggplant, trimmed
  and diced in $1/2$-inch pieces
1 teaspoon paprika
$1/4$ teaspoon nutmeg
$1/4$ teaspoon salt
6 plum tomatoes, chopped
$1\,1/2$ cups soybeans
$1/2$ cup bread crumbs

Preheat oven to 350 degrees. Sauté onion and garlic in olive oil for 1 minute. Add eggplant and sauté for 5 to 10 minutes or until eggplant is soft. Stir in paprika, nutmeg, and salt. Transfer contents of sauté pan to a $2\,1/2$-quart casserole dish. Add chopped tomatoes and soybeans and stir to combine. Sprinkle bread crumbs over the top. Bake casserole, covered, for 30 minutes. Uncover and bake 15 more minutes or until top is lightly browned.

CAULIFLOWER BEET CASSEROLE

This salad is absolutely beautiful! The white cauliflower turns a lovely shade of pink as it marinates with the beets. It is an easy dish to prepare and can be made well in advance. It is perfect for a buffet table or served as an hors d'oeuvre. For instructions on cooking beets, see the recipe for Tobee's Borscht in this chapter, or use prepared canned or frozen beets.

1 head cauliflower, cut into florets
2 cups cooked beets, cut into thick chunks
Juice of 1 lemon
Salt and freshly ground white pepper to taste

Put cauliflower florets into pot with water to cover. Bring to a boil and cook over moderate heat for 10 minutes, until tender but crunchy. In glass bowl, combine beets and cauliflower. Pour in lemon juice. Season with salt and pepper. Toss well and let marinate in refrigerator for several hours. Serve well chilled.

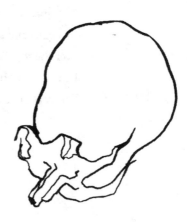

BAKED EGGPLANT CASSEROLE

2 eggplants, unpeeled
2 tablespoons olive oil
Juice of $1/2$ lemon
Salt and pepper
1 cup plain yogurt
1 large clove garlic, mashed
4 tablespoons minced scallion
2 tablespoons chopped parsley

Preheat oven to 350 degrees. Place eggplants on a baking sheet. Bake for 25 minutes or until tender. Remove from the oven and cool. Peel eggplants. Cut into large chunks and arrange in a nonstick shallow serving dish. Sprinkle with olive oil, lemon juice, salt, and pepper. Set aside. In a bowl, combine yogurt, garlic, and scallion. Toss eggplant with this dressing. Sprinkle with freshly chopped parsley. Chill well before serving.

STEAMED EGGPLANT

4 small whole eggplants, unpeeled
1 cup water
Salt
Paprika
Chives
Minced parsley

Steam small, whole, unpeeled eggplants above water until tender, for about 20 minutes. Split eggplants lengthwise and fluff the pulp with a fork. Season with salt, paprika, chives, and parsley. Spoon mixture back into eggplant shells. Serve hot.

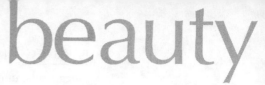

PURPLE DAY BEAUTY TREATMENT
Grapeseed Oil and Lavender

Today, discover two fantastic natural products that are
easy to find and easy to use: grapeseed oil and lavender.
Pure grapeseed oil, which can be found in most health-
food stores, is a great product to have around the house
for normal to dry skin. It rejuvenates the skin, hydrating thirsty skin surfaces. Moreover, grapeseed oil is a
wonderful antioxidant. It helps in fighting free radicals
from the environment that attack the skin. Massage it
into your legs, arms, hands and feet, even your face.

Grapeseed oil can be used on infants for massages.
Not only does it leave their skin feeling softer than ever,
but they also really love both the scent and texture of
the oil. If you have children, try using grapeseed oil for
chapped or rough skin, or for a calming massage before
bedtime.

A favorite natural product is lavender. Whether it is
cut right from the plant, dried and put into pouches, or
bought at the drugstore counter in the form of lavender
oil, lavender is one of the most beneficial natural products you can use. It gives our skin and bodies a wonderful boost.

Lavender can be used in small sachets to keep near the bed to cure bouts of insomnia. It not only eases the path to dream time, it also calms your skin and spirits. Lavender has both astringent and anti-inflammatory properties, helping to clear up breakouts, while soothing the skin. It is beneficial for all skin types.

If you are able to get some fresh lavender (many florists have it, and it can be ordered easily online), then soak a bunch of lavender herbs in warm water for at least two hours, overnight if possible. Once the water has been sufficiently infused with the lavender essence, soak a washcloth in the water for fifteen minutes, and then drape the washcloth over your eyes, neck, and face. The lavender will provide relief from exhaustion, as well as relaxing the muscles in the face. Try sprinkling it in your bath or adding lavender extract to your favorite moisturizer for a most calming effect.

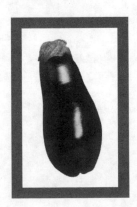

Yellow is sunshine and light, and you are entering a day of joy. Dance through these luscious foods, full of expectation and delight.

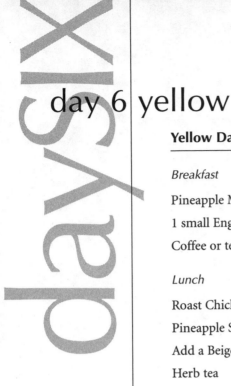

day 6 yellow

Yellow Day Sample Menu

Breakfast

Pineapple Milk Shake*

1 small English muffin

Coffee or tea

Lunch

Roast Chicken with Mustard and Herbs, 4 ounces*

Pineapple Squash, 1 cup*

Add a Beige

Herb tea

Snack

Banana with 1 tablespoon of peanut butter

Dinner

Lemon Consommé*

Israeli Baked Fish, 4 ounces*

Yellow and White Vegetable Casserole, 1 cup*

Yellow Day Bananas and Pineapple, 1 cup*

Decaffeinated coffee

Yellow Foods List

Yellow Fruits:
1 banana;
½ cup pineapple,
fresh or packed
in its own juice;
1 small golden
delicious apple;
lemons

Yellow Vegetables:
Unlimited amounts
of yellow squash,
wax beans

YELLOW DAY RECIPES

Yellow Salads and Luncheon Dishes

TROPICAL TUNA SALAD

Delicious luncheon dish.

1 8-ounce can white tuna, packed in water
1 slice fresh pineapple cut into chunks, or 1 8-ounce
   can pineapple chunks. (Reserve liquid.)
2 ribs celery, thinly sliced
$1/2$ cup water chestnuts, drained and sliced
2 tablespoons low-fat yogurt
2 tablespoons low-fat mayonnaise
1 tablespoon pineapple juice
Salt and pepper to taste

Drain tuna and break into chunks. Add pineapple,
celery, and water chestnuts. Mix yogurt, mayonnaise,
and juice and pour over tuna mixture. Cover tightly
and chill until ready to serve.

YELLOW DAY DIP

Delicious raw vegetable dip or salad dressing.

$1 1/4$ cups low-fat cottage cheese
$1/4$ cup pineapple chunks
$1/2$ cup unsweetened pineapple juice
1 clove garlic
1 teaspoon Vegit seasoning or seasoned salt
$1/8$ teaspoon freshly ground pepper

Put all ingredients in blender and puree until smooth.
Chill well. Makes 2 cups.

Yellow Soups

LEMON CONSOMMÉ

3 cups chicken broth
1/2 teaspoon grated lemon peel
2 tablespoons lemon juice
Lemon slices for each serving

Bring chicken broth to a boil. Add grated lemon peel and lemon juice. Pour into soup bowls and garnish each serving with a slice of lemon.

YELLOW SQUASH SOUP

1 tablespoon olive oil
4 scallions, minced
1 large clove garlic, minced
3 tablespoons minced parsley
2 cups coarsely chopped yellow squash
4 cups chicken stock
1 teaspoon salt
1/2 teaspoon pepper
1/2 teaspoon paprika
1 teaspoon caraway seeds
4 whole cloves
1 teaspoon sugar

Heat olive oil in soup pot. Sauté scallions, garlic, parsley, and squash for 2 minutes in the oil. Add chicken stock, salt, pepper, paprika, caraway seeds, cloves, and sugar. Cover and bring to boil on top of stove. Lower heat to simmer. Simmer covered for 20 minutes. Puree or serve as is. Serve hot.

Yellow Protein Dishes

LEMON FISH SAUTÉ

The simplest, tastiest way to serve fresh cod, haddock, sole, or flounder.

2 pounds fish fillets
1/4 cup fresh lemon juice
1 tablespoon olive oil
1/4 cup minced, fresh parsley
Lemon slices for garnish

In a glass bowl let fish marinate in lemon juice, turning once or twice, for 15 minutes. In nonstick skillet sauté fish in olive oil on each side until tender. Serve on warm platter with minced parsley and lemon slices.

ISRAELI BAKED FISH

2 small onions, chopped
2 teaspoons butter
2 pounds flounder fillets
2 tablespoons lemon juice
1/2 cup dry white wine
2 tablespoons minced parsley
1 cup sliced mushrooms
1/4 teaspoon salt
1/2 teaspoon pepper
Lemon slices for garnish

Preheat oven to 350 degrees. Sauté onion in butter in a nonstick skillet. Place flounder fillets on top of onions. Pour lemon juice and wine over fish. Sprinkle with parsley, mushrooms, salt, and pepper. Bake, covered, for 30 minutes. Serve hot. Garnish with lemon slices.

LEMON FISH MOUSSE

Yellow Day luncheon dish.

1 envelope unflavored gelatin
1 cup water
2 8-ounce cans of tuna, packed
   in water, drained and flaked
3/4 cup chopped celery
1/3 cup low-fat mayonnaise
1/4 cup chopped parsley
2 tablespoons lemon juice
1 teaspoon grated lemon peel
1 tablespoon grated onion
1 teaspoon celery seed
1 hard-boiled egg, minced

Sprinkle gelatin over water; heat, stirring until dissolved. Chill until slightly thickened. Combine gelatin with fish, celery, mayonnaise, parsley, lemon juice, lemon peel, onion, and celery seed. Pour into fish mold or glass bowl. Chill until well set. Garnish with parsley and chopped egg.

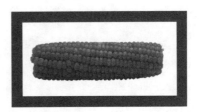

ROAST CHICKEN WITH MUSTARD AND HERBS

*This is an excellent way to prepare chicken
for the barbecue, as well.*

6 tablespoons prepared mustard
3 tablespoons minced shallots or scallions
$1/2$ teaspoon thyme, basil, or tarragon
$1/2$ teaspoon pepper
Two $2 1/2$-pound chickens, cut into serving pieces

Preheat oven to 375 degrees. Select an interesting mustard of the Dijon type. Try a lemon mustard or mustard with shallots. Blend mustard with shallots or onions, herbs, and pepper. "Paint" chicken with this mixture using a pastry brush. Arrange chicken pieces in a roasting pan and roast, uncovered, for 1 hour, or until tender. Place under broiler to brown slowly for 10 minutes on one side and 10 minutes on the other side. The chicken is done when the thickest part of the drumstick is pricked with a fork and the juices run clear yellow.

"The answer to dieting is not how little you eat, but how correctly you eat." The 7-Day Color Diet has helped show you how to eat correctly with a greater appreciation for fresh, natural foods. You have learned to eat a variety of foods that supply greater energy and promote better health.

LEMON OVEN-FRIED CHICKEN

2 chickens, cut into serving pieces
1 teaspoon salt
1 small onion, finely minced
1 teaspoon thyme, crushed
1 teaspoon marjoram, crushed
1 tablespoon grated lemon peel
2/3 cup lemon juice
1 cup water

Preheat oven to 400 degrees. Rub chicken with salt and arrange, skin side down, in a shallow baking dish. Mix onion, thyme, marjoram, lemon peel, juice, and water. Pour over chicken. Bake uncovered for 40 minutes. Turn chicken and bake 20 to 30 minutes longer, basting once or twice with pan drippings. Arrange chicken pieces on a warm platter and garnish with lemon slices.

Yellow Vegetables

PINEAPPLE SQUASH

4 cups thinly sliced yellow squash
1/2 small onion, finely grated
1 clove garlic, finely chopped
1/2 teaspoon salt
1/4 cup unsweetened pineapple juice
1/2 cup unsweetened pineapple chunks

Place squash, onion, garlic, salt, pineapple juice, and pineapple chunks in a covered saucepan. Bring to a boil. Reduce heat and simmer 10 minutes until squash is barely tender. Serve hot or cold.

YELLOW AND WHITE VEGETABLE CASSEROLE

1 head cauliflower, broken into florets
3 medium yellow squash, cut into chunks
2 cups water
Salt and pepper to taste
3 tablespoons minced parsley

Put 2 cups water in large pot with vegetable steamer inserted. Place cauliflower and squash on steamer rack. Bring water to boil. Cover pot and simmer for 15 minutes. Drain and refresh vegetables under cold water. Toss with salt, pepper, and minced parsley.

LEMON STEAMED CAULIFLOWER

Delicious hot or cold.

1 head cauliflower
$1/2$ cup lemon juice
1 cup water
1 teaspoon celery salt
1 teaspoon white pepper
Lemon slices for garnish

Wash cauliflower and break into florets. Toss with lemon juice and allow to marinate for $1/2$ hour. Steam cauliflower over vegetable steamer for 15 minutes, or until tender. Season cauliflower with celery salt and freshly ground white pepper. Garnish with lemon slices.

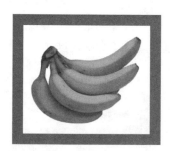

beauty

YELLOW DAY BEAUTY TREATMENT
Vitamin C

Perhaps the most important part of this great skin care rainbow is the Vitamin C that we get from fresh yellow and orange fruits, most notably from lemons. Vitamin C will tighten, brighten, and lighten your skin—great for both aging and sun-damaged skin. Vitamin C serums are recommended for all skin types, from dry to oily, because of the way in which Vitamin C strengthens the natural collagen in skin.

Vitamin C serves as a gentle exfoliant, ridding the skin of excess layers of dead skin. Nonetheless, it is very important to use all Vitamin C products precisely as directed on the label. Used correctly, Vitamin C products will have your skin looking younger and brighter than you ever thought possible. Physician's Choice of Arizona C-Quench Vitamin C Serum can be used for all skin types. Use it morning and night after cleansing. It prepares the skin to absorb whatever hydrating and moisturizing product you use.

This is the celebrate-all-colors day—the end of your first week on the 7-Day Color Diet. After Rainbow Day, you may repeat all the colors of the first week, then move on to the maintenance plan if you have met your weight loss goal. Do not stay on the 7-Day Color Diet for more than two weeks at a time without your doctor's approval.

Of course, the Rainbow Food List consists of all the foods from the other six Color Days. First here is the sample menu, then some wonderful recipes for celebrating all the colors.

day 7 rainbow

Rainbow Day Sample Menu

Breakfast

Pineapple-Strawberry Milk Shake*

Add a Beige

Coffee or tea

Lunch

Rainbow Chicken Salad, 4 ounces*

Rye bread, 1 slice

Herb tea

Snack

1 cup blueberries and sliced strawberries
mixed with cottage cheese

Dinner

Rainbow Gazpacho, 1 cup*

1 small baked potato with 2 ounces melted
low-fat cheddar cheese and broccoli

Orange-pineapple sherbet, 1 cup

Decaffeinated coffee

Rainbow Foods List

All the foods from the
other six Color Days.

RAINBOW DAY RECIPES

Rainbow Salads and Luncheon Dishes

RAINBOW SALAD NICOISE WITH VINAIGRETTE

Beautiful luncheon or light supper dish.

Serves 3.

3 cups cold, blanched string beans
3 quartered tomatoes
4 tablespoons vinaigrette dressing
1 head Boston lettuce, washed and dried
1 cup canned tuna chunks, packed
   in water, and drained
3 hard-boiled eggs, cold and cut into
   quarters (or 6 egg whites)
3 tablespoons minced, fresh green herbs

Just before serving, season beans and tomatoes with 2
tablespoons of vinaigrette. Toss lettuce leaves in the
salad bowl with 1 tablespoon vinaigrette and place
leaves around the edge of a bowl. Decorate the bowl
making layers of beans, tomatoes, tuna chunks, and
eggs. Pour remaining salad dressing over the salad and
sprinkle with herbs.

Vinaigrette
1 small clove garlic
1/2 teaspoon Dijon mustard
2 teaspoons lemon juice
2 tablespoons white wine vinegar
2 tablespoons safflower oil
Freshly ground pepper

Mash garlic. Add mustard and lemon juice. Mix well.
Add vinegar, oil, and pepper. Makes enough for one
large salad.

RAINBOW CHICKEN SALAD

The following dish is delicious. Tuna or turkey is just as good as the chicken.

Serves 4.

2 cups cold, cooked chicken, cut into chunks
2 cups fresh pineapple, or 1 15-ounce can
    pineapple chunks
1 rib celery, sliced
1/2 cucumber, peeled, seeded, and thickly sliced
1/2 green pepper, coarsely chopped
8 small mushrooms, thinly sliced
2 scallions, thinly sliced
1/2 cup low-fat mayonnaise
1 teaspoon curry powder

In large bowl toss together chicken, pineapple, celery, cucumber, green pepper, mushrooms, and scallions. In small bowl mix together mayonnaise and curry powder. Pour over salad. Toss well. Serve well chilled.

PURPLE CABBAGE AND ZUCCHINI SLAW WITH CELERY SEED DRESSING

Serves 8.

1 large head purple cabbage, shredded
2 large zucchini, thinly sliced
3 scallions, thinly sliced
1/4 cup minced parsley

Combine all ingredients and toss with
Celery Seed Dressing.

Celery Seed Dressing

1/2 cup low-fat mayonnaise
1 tablespoon celery seed
1 garlic clove, minced
1 teaspoon white pepper
2 teaspoons Dijon mustard
1 tablespoon fresh dill, or 1 teaspoon dried
3 tablespoons red wine vinegar

Whip up ingredients in blender or food processor and
pour over salad 30 minutes before serving. Chill well.

MOMEE'S LECHO

*This is a Hungarian luncheon dish that is still my favorite
way to prepare eggs.*

Serves 4.

1 tablespoon oil
1 small onion, chopped
1 small green pepper, chopped
1 cup sliced mushrooms
2 tomatoes, chopped
1/4 cup water
6 eggs (or 10 egg whites),
    or 1 cup egg substitute (Eggbeaters)

Put oil in nonstick skillet. Brown onions.

Add green pepper, mushrooms, tomatoes,

and water. Cook vegetables, covered, on low heat until soft, about 15 minutes. In separate dish lightly scramble eggs and pour over vegetables, continuing to scramble in the skillet, uncovered. Season to taste with some salt and pepper. Serve immediately.

Rainbow Soups

BERKELEY RAINBOW SOUP

I was inspired to include this recipe by my friend Gail Berland who always understood the beauty of the understated. This soup is excellent made in advance and reheated.

Serves 8.

8 well-ripened tomatoes
1 cup sliced onions
1 tablespoon olive oil
1 clove garlic, crushed
$1/2$ cup minced scallions, white and green parts
2 stalks celery, thinly sliced
2 large carrots, cut in thin rounds
2 tablespoons flour
8 cups chicken stock
3 tablespoons tomato paste
1 cup tomato juice
$1/2$ teaspoon dried basil
6 peppercorns
Salt to taste

Peel and seed tomatoes and cut into quarters. In soup pot, sauté the onions in oil. Add tomatoes and garlic and stir until tomato juices have evaporated. Add scallions, celery, and carrots. Stir for 5 minutes. Sprinkle in flour and stir for 3 minutes. Pour in 2 cups of the stock and stir until smooth. Add tomato paste, tomato juice, rest of stock, basil, peppercorns, and salt. Stir well. Cover and simmer, stirring often, for 45 minutes.

RAINBOW DILL SOUP

Serves 8.

1 tablespoon olive oil
1/2 cup finely chopped onions
1/2 cup coarsely chopped celery
1 large carrot, cut in 1/8-inch rounds
1 16-ounce can peeled tomatoes
1 quart chicken stock
1/2 teaspoon salt
Freshly ground pepper to taste
1 1/2 to 2 teaspoons dried dill
1/2 cup fresh green beans, cut into 2-inch pieces
1/2 medium-sized cauliflower, cut into florets

In a large pot, heat olive oil over moderate heat. Add onions, celery, and carrots, and sauté, stirring about 8 minutes. Do not brown onions. Add canned tomatoes with juice, chicken stock, salt, and pepper. Cover pot and bring to a boil over high heat. Reduce heat to low and simmer 25 minutes. Add dill, beans, and cauliflower. Return to boil, reduce heat, and simmer 15 minutes more or until vegetables are barely tender; avoid overcooking. Serve hot.

RAINBOW GAZPACHO I

Serves 8.

2 cucumbers, peeled, seeded, and cubed
1 green pepper, seeded and sliced
2 stalks celery, diced
1 medium onion, diced
1 1-pound can stewed tomatoes,
   or 4 to 6 fresh, peeled tomatoes, cut up
2 tablespoons red wine vinegar
1 tablespoon lemon juice
1/2 teaspoon Tabasco sauce
1/2 teaspoon Worcestershire sauce
1 teaspoon salt
1 teaspoon pepper
2 tablespoons minced parsley

Place all ingredients in blender, about $1/3$ at a time, and blend each batch for 10 seconds. Chill several hours. Garnish with chopped cucumber and minced parsley.

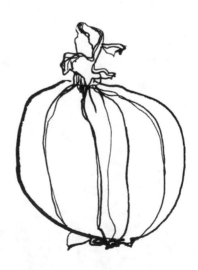

RAINBOW GAZPACHO II

*This recipe, given to me by Betty and Izzy Schreiber,
is my favorite summer soup.*

Serves 6.

2 large tomatoes, peeled and halved
1 large cucumber
1 medium onion, peeled and halved
1 medium green pepper, quartered
1 jar pimento, drained
2 12-ounce cans tomato juice, well chilled
1 tablespoon olive oil
2 tablespoons red wine vinegar
$1/8$ teaspoon Tabasco sauce
$1^1/2$ teaspoons salt and dash black pepper
1 garlic clove (optional)
Chives and lemon slices (optional)

In blender, place 1 large tomato, half of cucumber, half
of onion, 1 pepper quarter, the pimento, and $1/2$ cup of
tomato juice. Puree at high speed for 30 seconds. In
bowl mix pureed vegetables with remaining juice, oil,
vinegar, Tabasco sauce, salt, and black pepper.
Refrigerate, covered, at least 2 hours. Before serving stir
the crushed garlic clove through soup if desired. Chop
remaining vegetables to serve with soup. Garnish with
chives and thin lemon slices.

FISH CHOWDER

Serves 6.

4 cups water
2 onions, chopped
1 clove garlic, minced
2 cups tomatoes, peeled and seeded
2 stalks celery, diced
2 carrots, diced
1 bay leaf, crumbled
1/4 teaspoon fennel seed
1 teaspoon pepper
1/2 teaspoon thyme
1/4 teaspoon saffron
2 tablespoons minced parsley
2 teaspoons salt
1/2 teaspoon savory
2 pounds fresh fish—large chunks of halibut,
   sole, haddock
2 tablespoons lemon juice

Put all ingredients except fish and lemon juice in a large
soup pot. Bring to boil. Add fish and lemon juice.
Lower heat. Cover and simmer for 30 minutes. Season
with salt and pepper to taste.

Rainbow Fish Dishes

RAINBOW BAKED FISH

Serves 3.

2 stalks celery, diced
2 carrots, sliced
1 onion, sliced
2 tomatoes, coarsely chopped
1 pound fish fillets (sole, haddock, or flounder)
1 teaspoon salt
$1/2$ teaspoon pepper
1 tablespoon paprika
1 teaspoon fresh dill

Preheat oven to 350 degrees. Combine celery, carrots, onion, and tomatoes. Line roasting pan with vegetable mixture. Place fish on top of vegetables. Sprinkle with salt, pepper, paprika, and dill. Bake, covered, for 30 minutes.

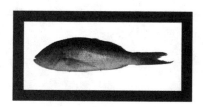

Rainbow Chicken Dishes

LOIS'S RAINBOW CHICKEN

This Indian dish was given to me by my friend Lois Steinitz, who is a constant inspiration for staying healthy and slim. The dish is mild, colorful, and easy to make.

Serves 4.

One 2^1/2-pound chicken, cut into serving pieces
1 teaspoon salt
Freshly ground pepper
1 onion, chopped
1 green pepper, chopped
1 clove garlic, minced
2 teaspoons curry powder
^{1}/2 teaspoon coriander
^{1}/2 teaspoon turmeric
^{1}/2 teaspoon thyme
1 16-ounce can of tomatoes, with liquid

Preheat oven to 350 degrees. Season chicken with salt and pepper. In a nonstick skillet brown chicken on all sides. Remove chicken from skillet and add onion, green pepper, garlic, curry powder, coriander, turmeric, and thyme. Cook until onion wilts. Add tomatoes with the liquid and stir well. Return the chicken to the skillet, skin side up. Cover tightly and bake for 1^1/2 hours.

RAINBOW ROAST CHICKEN

This is my favorite way of preparing roast chicken.

Serves 4 to 6.

1 3-pound chicken, cut into serving pieces
Salt, pepper, and paprika
2 carrots, peeled and quartered
1 large onion, coarsely chopped
1 large green pepper, cut into strips
2 ribs celery, cut into large chunks
1/2 cup minced fresh parsley

Preheat oven to 350 degrees. Season chicken well with
salt, pepper, and paprika. In large roasting pan make
a bed of the carrots, onion, green pepper, and celery.
Place chicken on vegetables and sprinkle with parsley.
Bake, uncovered, for 45 minutes and covered for
30 minutes.

Rainbow Vegetables

COLD DISH OF ZUCCHINI AND
TOMATOES WITH GARLIC AND LEMON

Delicious as a first course, hors d'oeuvre, or side dish.

Serves 4 to 6.

2 pounds zucchini
1 pound small, ripe tomatoes
2 large cloves garlic, peeled and minced
2 tablespoons lemon juice
1 tablespoon fresh tarragon or 1 1/2 teaspoons dried
Salt
Freshly ground black pepper
1 large lemon

Peel zucchini and cut into 1-inch slices. Peel and seed
tomatoes and chop roughly. In an enameled skillet put
the zucchini, tomatoes, minced garlic, lemon juice, and

half of the herbs. Season with salt and pepper. Stir, bring to boil, and let simmer uncovered until the zucchini are tender, about 25 minutes. Peel the lemon, remove seeds, and chop the pulp. Add lemon to vegetables when they have completed cooking. Let cool. When cold, sprinkle with remaining herbs and refrigerate. Chill well. Can be made several days in advance.

RAINBOW STIR-FRY VEGETABLES

Serves 2.

2 teaspoons vegetable oil or olive oil
$1/2$ cup slivered carrots
$1/2$ cup slivered celery
1 medium zucchini, thinly sliced
2 tablespoons chicken broth or water
Salt, pepper to taste

Put oil in nonstick skillet and bring to high heat. Add carrots and stir-fry for 1 minute. Add celery and zucchini and stir 1 minute. Add chicken broth or water and cover. Cook 1 minute. Season with salt and pepper.

GREEN BEANS IN BASIL SAUCE

This delicious vegetable dish can be served cold. Excellent as a side dish to grilled fish or chicken.

Serves 4.

1 pound fresh green beans
2 teaspoons olive oil
1 medium onion, thinly sliced
4 ripe tomatoes, peeled, seeded, and chopped
Salt and white pepper
1 bay leaf
1/2 cup finely chopped fresh basil,
    or 2 teaspoons dried
2 garlic cloves
1/4 cup parsley

Snap off the tips of the green beans. Steam beans until crisp (10 minutes). Drain and rinse under cold water to refresh. In a large skillet heat olive oil. Add onion and cook for 10 minutes, covered, over low heat, until tender. Add tomatoes, salt, pepper, and bay leaf. Cook the mixture for 10 minutes over high heat until very thick. Remove bay leaf. Add drained green beans to the skillet and simmer, covered, for 5 minutes. Puree the basil, garlic, and parsley in a blender. Add the puree to the tomato and bean mixture. Heat through and serve.

beauty

RAINBOW DAY BEAUTY TREATMENT
Repeat What Feels Best and "Add a Beige"
Oatmeal Bath or Clay Mask

Once you have experienced the full benefit of the 7-Day Color Cure, you will be able to evaluate what else your skin type needs. If your skin benefited from the cucumber or lavender treatment, then indulge in both today. Feel free to "Add a Beige" and take an oatmeal bath or use a clay mask. Experiment with what feels best! After a while, you will develop a routine that your skin will love. Some products, like the Vitamin C serums and papain enzymes, will take longer than a week to show results. But do not fret, using these natural and effective treatments will help you maintain a healthy and balanced complexion.

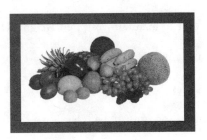

CHAPTER 11

The Color Diet Weight Maintenance Plan

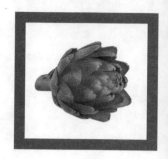

For good health, be sure you eat a variety of foods daily, with an emphasis on the less fatty foods.

Dr. Morton B. Glen, in his book *But I Don't Eat That Much*, says, "The answer to dieting is not how little you eat, but how correctly you eat." The 7-Day Color Diet has helped show you how to eat correctly with a greater appreciation for fresh, natural foods. You have learned to eat a variety of foods that supply greater energy and promote better health.

So what happens now that you have reached your goal and want to maintain your new weight? Obviously, you do not want to limit yourself to "one-color days" for the rest of your life. By following the Color Diet Maintenance Program you will develop a controlled system of eating that will help you stay slim and healthy.

It is important to continue to eat well and select widely from a variety of foods. Reverting to old eating choices means a return to patterns and foods that made you unhealthy to begin with.

Always keep in mind that there is not any one food that can make you fat. The only way to put on weight is to take in more calories than your body uses up. More calories of anything—too much cottage cheese, for example—can mean extra calories and additional weight.

Learn to taste and enjoy everything—but in moderation. Eat only what you enjoy and only when you are hungry.

Should you notice a weight gain, as we all do from time to time, go back on White Day immediately. After a day or two on it, you will lose the extra weight. You don't ever want the pounds to accumulate again. You now know the divine joy of being a slender person. "Nothing tastes as good as slim feels."

Maintenance Plan Menu Allowances

Breakfast

1 fruit or ³/4 cup juice

1 cup nonfat milk

1 slice whole wheat bread, or 1 cup unsweetened cereal

1 egg (limited to 4 per week)

Lunch

One serving chosen from the following proteins:

- 4 ounces fish or shellfish
- 4 ounces chicken or turkey
- 4 ounces tofu
- 1 cup cottage cheese
- 2 cups plain nonfat yogurt
  (1 cup may be used in soup, dressing, or dessert)
- 2 eggs (limited to 4 per week)
- 2 ounces hard cheese

Plus:

2 cups raw vegetable salad

1 fruit

1 small bagel, English muffin, or 2 slices bread*

*Beware of "deli-size" bagels. Always opt for
single-serving, presliced frozen ones.

Dinner

One serving chosen from the following proteins:

- 4 ounces fish or shellfish
- 4 ounces chicken or turkey
- 4 ounces beef, lamb, or veal
- 1 cup legumes or 4 ounces tofu or tempeh

Plus:

1 cup raw vegetable salad

1 cup cooked vegetables

1 fruit

Additional Daily Allowances:

2 tablespoons mayonnaise, oil, butter, or margarine

1 glass of skim milk

1 small baked potato, or 1 cup brown rice

1 cup brown rice

1 cup whole wheat pasta

1/2 whole wheat bagel

1 whole wheat English muffin

1 slice whole wheat, rye, or pumpernickel bread

Unlimited white vegetables

Unlimited herb tea, decaffeinated coffee, diet soda

Unlimited herbs, spices, mustard,
  wine vinegar, lemon juice

Sample Menu

Breakfast

Orange juice, 1 cup

Whole wheat toast, 1 slice

Scrambled egg, 1

Nonfat milk, 8 ounces (plain or as a milk shake)

Coffee or tea

Lunch

Rainbow Chicken Salad, 4 ounces*

Small toasted bagel, 1

Orange Day Coleslaw, 1 cup*

Cantaloupe, 1

Herb tea

Dinner

Rainbow Dill Soup, 1 cup*

Hungarian Baked Fish, 4 ounces*

Marinated Carrot Casserole, $1/2$ cup*

1 cup freshly steamed broccoli

1 cup orange pineapple sherbet

Coffee or tea

ENTERTAINING

There was a time when if "company" were coming, I went to great lengths to prepare especially rich, delicious, and, usually, fattening dishes. I used company as an excuse to indulge in foods that left me feeling fat and guilty once my guests left. For a while, I stopped entertaining altogether. I was always waiting to be off my diet. I felt terribly deprived.

I have since learned that it is possible both to entertain and to serve a lovely meal without putting on weight. If you enjoy entertaining and feeding your friends and family well, learn to take pride in serving a colorful, healthy meal rather than a fattening one.

For example, try a menu of a tossed salad of crisp green lettuce and sliced tomatoes with a light French vinaigrette to start, followed by Green Day Roast Chicken, freshly steamed lemon broccoli, and bright

It is possible both to entertain and to serve a lovely meal without putting on weight. If you enjoy entertaining and feeding your friends and family well, learn to take pride in serving a colorful, healthy meal rather than a fattening one.

orange-glazed carrots. For dessert, bake a hot apple-pineapple pie in a pie plate without a crust. It is a lovely, light meal; and whenever I serve it, I receive as many compliments as I did for any high calorie menu from the bad old days.

It is very simple to orchestrate a meal that is as beautiful to look at as it is to eat. Take advantage of what is fresh and in season. In the spring, a favorite luncheon is grilled salmon and lightly steamed asparagus. In the winter, it is a hot vegetable soup made of chunks of carrots, celery, and mushrooms.

Vary your desserts by season as well. In the winter, I like to serve hot baked apples sprinkled with cinnamon. In summer, I offer bowls of fresh, red berries topped with cool yogurt and honey.

Wisely invest the time you spend feeding your friends and family. Plan a colorful meal that will delight the senses. Combine a variety of textures and flavors. Use your energy not in baking a rich cake that everyone will hate you for when they climb on the scales the next morning, but in making a light, fun dessert like Red Berries Romanoff instead.

You don't have to deprive yourself of the pleasure of sharing an evening of food with friends, just make it with the right foods. Let it be a colorful, tasty meal rather than a fattening one. And remember, your over-weight friends may want to get thinner and your slim friends want to stay that way. Serve a light meal and everyone will be happy.

EATING OUT

Eating out, whether in a restaurant or at a friend's home, should not present a problem. At a restaurant there is always a variety of foods to choose from. Ask for foods prepared exactly as you like them. If you don't like your salads or entrees swimming in rich sauces, ask for the dressings and sauces to be served on the side. Dip your fork in the dressing before you spear the salad to limit your intake of the dressing. Ask for your veg-etables to be served fresh, without butter. People in the restaurant business are there to serve you.

There is no reason in the world not to eat out. You can have a wonderful time without putting on weight. Have dessert, but let it be the right dessert for you. Choose from the fresh fruits in season. Red raspberries, sweet strawberries, and fresh melons are usually available in most restaurants and are very satisfying. If you do not see these foods listed on the dessert section of the menu, check under appetizers. If you do want to indulge in a rich dessert on a special occasion, don't deprive yourself! Pick something you really love, savor it, and eat it sparingly.

When you are at someone's home for a meal, don't allow yourself to feel trapped because you don't have control over what is being served. No matter what is served, no matter how rich the meal, tell yourself that if you just eat half of it you will do fine. You will enjoy the meal without feeling guilty.

And always, no matter where you are, eat slowly. Savor every mouthful. Eating well is an art. Enjoy it.

BINGEING

How often do you pace the kitchen, opening and closing the refrigerator and pantry doors, over and over again, hoping to find something to "munch" on? And how often, if you find something like a box of cookies or a pint of ice cream, do you proceed to finish the whole thing while wondering, "Why am I doing this?" Compulsive eating and bingeing is destructive behavior.

We all know that we don't always eat because we are hungry. We often eat because we are anxious, tired, bored, angry, frustrated, and so on. We eat to avoid having to deal with feelings or we eat to feed our emotions. But the truth is that the only thing that really gets fed at those times are our hips.

I am convinced that there are some of us who, even with years of therapy and all the behavior modification techniques available, will forever want to eat in response to stress, whether it be good stress or bad stress. Dr. Frank J. Bruno, a psychologist who deals with problems of overweight, writes in his book, *Think Yourself Thin*, that overeating is due most often to an intense oral craving. At these times, it is absolutely necessary to put something in one's mouth. The trick, he claims, is to teach yourself to reach for something non-fattening in order to stay slim. The truth is we do not taste what we are eating in response to emotional stress. The secret is to get through that period of emotional stress without getting fat. It is enough having to cope with the feelings, without adding extra anxiety and guilt for overeating.

Let's talk rationally for a minute. After all, at the moment you feel like bingeing, you are not in a position to think creatively about how to get through that awful compulsion to eat. It is now, during a moment of peace, that the problem should be thought through. It is helpful to have a solution on hand for when the crazy attack hits.

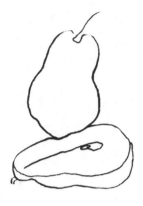

I, and many others who have managed to stay slim, have found it very helpful to always have raw vegetables on hand, white ones in particular. Mushrooms, cauliflower, coleslaw, and bean sprouts should always be ready to grab. They can be eaten plain, lightly steamed, or raw with a light dressing. Have them on hand and learn to reach for them when you absolutely must have something. It is a positive way to deal with compulsive eating. Some experts in the field of overeating feel it is best not to reach for anything. I am convinced these experts have never been hit by a compulsive eating attack. There has to be something there to reach for. Plan for it now and you won't be left consuming a box of cookies that, after the first bite, you cease to taste anyhow. That way, when the need to binge is over, you will still like yourself.

Don't be too hard on yourself when you do give in to a binge. We all do it. It doesn't mean that you will never get slim, or stay that way once you've reached your goal. All it means is that you will have to "pay for it." You will have to be a bit stricter at the next meal or the next day so that your body can burn up the extra calories you consumed during your binge. Within a day or two your weight will be back to normal.

One final word on bingeing. Many years ago, I read an article discussing compulsive eating. One woman said that when she starts a binge she just can't stop. She feels she has a license to eat the rest of the day or night. The psychologist who wrote the article suggested that at such times you should remember that just because you put a dent in your car doesn't mean you have to go ahead and demolish the whole thing. That thought has helped me through many an almost-binge.

Remember—if you have lost control, you simply were not prepared for the situation and your reaction to it. The worst thing you can do is to label yourself. The best thing you can do is to think things through and resolve to be better prepared the next time.

THE 7-DAY COLOR DIET CALORIE GUIDE

We don't believe in counting calories, but we do believe in monitoring your portions. We realize, however, that many people feel more comfortable with calories. If so, here's a quick reference guide. It also gives recommended portions for each food type, so you can control your intake.

White Foods

	Quantity	Calories
Dairy Products		
Butter	1 tablespoon	100
Buttermilk	1 cup	90
Cottage cheese, creamed	1 cup	240
	1 tablespoon	16
Cottage cheese	1 cup	195
Cream cheese	1 ounce	105
	1 tablespoon	50
Jarlsberg cheese	1 ounce	95
Monterey Jack cheese	1 ounce	100
Muenster cheese	1 ounce	100
Swiss cheese	1 ounce	90
Cream, half and half	1 cup	325
	1 tablespoon	20
Cream, light whipping	1 tablespoon	45
Cream, heavy whipping	1 tablespoon	55
Eggs	1 large	75
Eggs, white	1	15
Eggs, yolk	1	60
Margarine	1 tablespoon	100
Mayonnaise	1 tablespoon	100
Oil, salad and cooking	1 tablespoon	105
Yogurt, nonfat (plain)	1 cup	120
	1 tablespoon	10
Fruit		
White grapefruit	1 cup	55
White grapes, seedless	1 cup	95
Fruit juices		
Grapefruit juice	1 cup	95
Vegetables		
Bean sprouts	1 cup	4
Cabbage	1 head	60
Cauliflower, cooked	1 cup	25
Cauliflower, raw	1 cup	14
Endive	1 cup	10

Mushrooms	1 large	10
Mushrooms, canned	1 cup	40
Mushrooms, chopped	1 cup	64
Onions, raw	1	40
Parsnips, cooked	1 cup	100
Water chestnuts	1	6

Fish

Flounder, raw	3 ounces	66
Haddock, raw	3 ounces	67
Halibut, raw	3 ounces	85
Trout	3 ounces	170
Tuna	3 ounces	125

Chicken

| Breast, broiled without skin | 3 ounces | 120 |
| Dark meat, without skin | 3 ounces | 160 |

Red Foods

Fruits

Apples, raw	1 medium	80
Applesauce, unsweetened	1 cup	70
Apricots, raw	3 medium	55
packed in own juice	1 cup	50
Cranberries, raw	1 cup	100
Grapefruit (pink)	1 medium	60
Raspberries	1/2 cup	45
Rhubarb	1 cup	19
Strawberries	1 cup	55
Watermelon	4 x 8-inch wedge	115

Fruit juices

Apple juice	1 cup	120
Cranberry juice	1 cup	160
Grapefruit juice, fresh	1 cup	45
canned, sweetened	1/2 cup	130

Vegetables

Cabbage, red	1 cup	25
Peppers, red	1 pod	20
Pimento	1 medium jar	10
Radishes	4 small	5
Sweet potatoes	1 cup cooked	155
Tomatoes	1 medium	35

Vegetable juices

Tomato juice	1 cup	45
V-8 juice	1 cup	35

Fish

Red snapper	3 ounces	100
Shrimp	1 large	25
Lobster, canned	1 cup	75

Green Foods

Fruits

Apple, green	1 medium	70
Green grapes	1 cup	95
Honeydew	1/4 melon or 1 cup	50
Pear, raw	1 medium	80

Fruit juices

Lime juice	1 tablespoon	4

Vegetables

Artichokes	1 French or globe	50
	4 small Jerusalem	70
	1 bottom	25
Asparagus	1 cup cooked	35
	6 canned spears	20
Avocado	1	180
Beans, green snap	1 cup	25
Beans, lima, cooked	1 cup	180
Broccoli spears	1 cup	45
Brussels sprouts, cooked	1 cup	45
Cabbage, green	1 head	60
Celery	1 cup, diced	15
	1 large stalk	30
Chard	1 cup steamed	30
Collards, leaves and stalks	1 cup	51
Cucumber	1 raw	30
Green pepper	1 large	25
Peas, fresh	1 cup	110
Peas, canned	1 cup	130
Kohlrabi, raw, sliced	1 cup	40
Lettuce, Boston	1 head	30
Lettuce, iceberg	1 head	60
Scallions, green	1 small	4
Spinach, cooked	1 cup	40
Spinach, raw, chopped	1 cup	10

Sprouts—all varieties	$1/4$ cup	4
Watercress	1 cup	4
Zucchini	1 cup	46

Orange Foods

Fruits

Apricots, fresh	3 medium	55
Apricots, dried	4 halves	40
Cantaloupe	$1/2$	60
Orange	1 medium	65
Peach, fresh	1 medium	35
Tangerine	1 medium	40
Nectarine	1 medium	40

Fruit juices

| Orange juice | 1 cup | 112 |
| Peach nectar | 1 cup | 120 |

Fish

| Salmon | 4 ounces | 150 |

Vegetables

Carrots	1 whole	20
Carrots, grated	1 cup	45
Carrots, diced, cooked	1 cup	45

Cheeses

Cheddar	1 ounce	100
Cheddar, grated	1 tablespoon	30
American cheese	1 ounce	100

Purple Foods

Fruits

Blackberries	1 cup	85
Blueberries	1 cup	85
Plums, fresh	1 medium	25
	3 canned	100
Prunes, dried, pitted	4 medium	70
	1 cup cooked	100
Purple grapes	1 cup	65

Fruit juices

| Grape juice | 1 cup | 165 |
| Prune juice | 1 cup | 200 |

Vegetables

Beets, cooked, diced	1 cup	50
Eggplant, cooked	1 cup	22
Purple cabbage	1 cup shredded	25
	1 head	60

Yellow Foods

Fruits

Banana	1 small	85
Pineapple, fresh, diced	1 cup	75
Pineapple, canned	2 small slices	90

Fruit juices

Pineapple juice	1 cup	135

Vegetables

Squash, summer, fresh	1 cup	30
Squash, yellow, frozen	1 cup	40
Wax beans	1 cup	45

Miscellaneous

Breads and Grains

Bagel	1	75
Bread crumbs	1/4 cup	50
Cracked wheat bread	1 slice	55
English muffin	1	75
Rye bread, thin	1 slice	55
Whole wheat bread	1 slice	60

Cereals

Wheat flakes	1 ounce	100
Wheat germ	1 tablespoon	15
Whole wheat flour	1 tablespoon	25
	1 cup	400

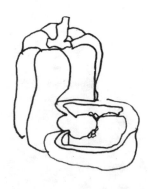

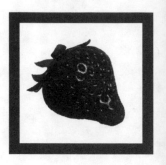

CHAPTER 12

Treat Yourself

When you are trying to lose weight on the 7-Day Color
Diet, it's best to stick to fresh fruits, prepared simply
and without adornment. Learn to savor the natural,
sweet flavor of fresh seasonal fruits. A cold slice of
melon or a hot, baked apple can take care of any
sweet tooth.

But when you are entertaining or have reached the
maintenance stage of the 7-Day Color Diet, you can
treat yourself to the desserts in this chapter. These
recipes are both low in calories and absolutely delicious
dessert treats.

It really is okay to have dessert, just make sure it is
the right kind. Make dessert worth eating—luscious as
well as nourishing. And, as always, be creative. Combine
fruits of all colors, flavors, and textures for a rainbow of
eating pleasure.

A RAINBOW OF DESSERT TREATS

HOT SPICED PEARS

This is a favorite fall dessert. It is also delicious when served cold.

4 firm, ripe pears, peeled, halved, and cored
2 cups cider or apple juice
1 teaspoon cinnamon
4 cloves

In a large skillet combine pears, cider, cinnamon, and cloves. Cook gently over low heat, covered, for 20 to 25 minutes. Remove from the cooking liquid and serve warm in pretty dessert dishes with the liquid spooned over it.

CURRIED FRESH PEARS

3 pears, peeled, halved, and cored
1 tablespoon butter
2 tablespoons brown sugar
1 teaspoon curry powder
$1/4$ teaspoon salt
$1/4$ cup dry white wine

Preheat oven to 350 degrees. Place pears in baking dish. In small bowl make a paste of butter, brown sugar, curry, and salt. Fill cavity of each pear with some of this mixture. Pour wine over pears. Cover loosely with aluminum foil. Bake until tender, 30 to 40 minutes.

RED DAY APPLESAUCE

This is excellent hot or cold.

8 cups peeled and cored apple slices
2 cups water
1 tablespoon lemon juice
1 teaspoon cinnamon
1 teaspoon nutmeg
1 tablespoon honey

In a 6-quart kettle place apple slices, water, and lemon juice. Bring to a boil and simmer until almost soft (10 minutes). Add cinnamon, nutmeg, and honey. Puree in a food mill or blender.

BAKED APPLES

6 large apples, peeled halfway down and cored
1 teaspoon honey for each apple
Cinnamon
Nutmeg
2 cups boiling water or apple juice

Preheat oven to 400 degrees. In a baking dish, arrange the apples with the peeled ends up. Fill each cavity with honey and sprinkle with cinnamon and nutmeg. Cover the bottom of the dish with boiling water or juice. Bake the apples, uncovered, for 30 minutes or until tender. Baste them often with pan juices.

RED BERRIES ROMANOFF

2 cups plain low-fat yogurt
2 tablespoons honey
1 1/2 teaspoons vanilla extract
4 cups fresh strawberries or raspberries

Mix yogurt with honey and vanilla. Chill dressing until ready to serve. Spoon berries into dessert dishes and top with yogurt dressing.

CINNAMON BROILED GRAPEFRUIT

1 grapefruit, halved
$1/2$ teaspoon cinnamon
1 teaspoon granulated brown sugar

Preheat broiler. Loosen sections of grapefruit. Combine cinnamon and brown sugar. Sprinkle on grapefruit halves. Place in preheated broiler for 5 minutes. Serve hot and bubbling.

ORANGE PINEAPPLE SHERBET

This is a light and refreshing dessert any time of year.

1 6-ounce can undiluted
   frozen orange juice concentrate
1 20-ounce can unsweetened
   pineapple in its own juice
1 cup skim milk

Combine ingredients in blender, mixing on low speed for 10 seconds. Pour into $1^1/2$-quart mold. Place in freezer overnight. Allow to soften slightly before serving. Garnish with orange slices.

WINTER SHERBET

Prepare at least 8 hours before serving.

Two $8^1/2$-ounce cans crushed pineapple, packed
   in its own juice
One 16-ounce can peaches, packed in their own juice
2 tablespoons lemon juice
$1/4$ teaspoon vanilla extract

In food processor or electric blender, blend pineapple, peaches, and juice from both cans until smooth. Stir in lemon juice and vanilla. Freeze this mixture until mushy, stirring occasionally. In 2 hours, blend mixture again until smooth ($1/3$ of mixture at a time). Freeze until the consistency of sherbet. Thaw at room temperature 5 minutes before serving.

HONEYED FRUIT YOGURT

Easy. Can be made in advance.

16 ounces nonfat plain yogurt
2 tablespoons honey
1 orange, peeled and cut into bite-sized pieces
8 ounces crushed pineapple, juice pack, drained

Mix yogurt and honey until smooth. Add orange sections and crushed pineapple. Chill overnight.

ORANGES IN RED WINE

$\frac{1}{2}$ cup dry red wine
1 tablespoon honey
1 cinnamon stick
2 cloves
$\frac{1}{2}$ lemon, thinly sliced
Peel of 1 orange
2 to 3 large oranges, thinly sliced

Put wine, honey, cinnamon stick, cloves, and lemon slices in saucepan and bring to a boil. Reduce heat and simmer 5 minutes. Peel oranges, reserving skin. Cut the peel into thin strips. Cut peeled oranges into thin slices and put into a square glass dish. Pour hot syrup over oranges. Sprinkle orange peel on top. Chill until ready to serve.

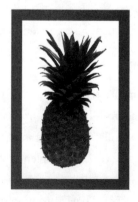

GINGERED BLUEBERRY COMPOTE

1 cup orange juice
1 tablespoon lemon juice
1 tablespoon honey
1 teaspoon grated fresh ginger
1 pint fresh or frozen blueberries

Combine orange juice, lemon juice, honey, and ginger.
Place blueberries in an attractive glass bowl and pour
orange juice mixture over them. Serve immediately.

BAKED BANANAS AND BLUEBERRIES

6 bananas, peeled, sliced lengthwise
1 cup fresh blueberries
1 tablespoon brown sugar
1 cup orange juice

Preheat oven to 350 degrees. Place bananas in a baking
dish. Sprinkle blueberries and brown sugar over
bananas and then pour orange juice over the fruit. Heat
30 minutes or until bubbling. Delicious hot, and good
served cold with a dollop of yogurt on top.

YELLOW DAY BANANAS AND PINEAPPLE

*This is a delicious dessert to be made right before serving.
Save some fruit from your morning milk shake for this.*

4 slices pineapple, fresh or canned in its own juices
2 medium bananas, sliced
1/2 cup nonfat yogurt
1 tablespoon honey
2 teaspoons lemon or lime juice

Divide pineapple and bananas into four dessert dishes.
Mix yogurt with honey and lemon or lime juice. Pour
over sliced pineapple and bananas.

HOT APRICOT SOUFFLÉ

The fruit in this recipe must be well drained. The drier the puree, the lighter the soufflé will be. This light and tasty soufflé can be made with canned peaches as well.

1 28-ounce can apricot halves,
   packed in their own juice, drained
Dash of salt
Lemon juice
1 tablespoon sugar
4 egg whites, beaten to stiff peaks

Preheat oven to 350 degrees. Puree apricots in blender or food processor. Pour into saucepan. Add salt, lemon juice, and sugar. Simmer puree for 5 minutes, stirring constantly. Fold the puree into the beaten egg whites. Spray a soufflé dish lightly with a low-calorie oil spray. Pour the mixture into dish and bake for 30 minutes or until well puffed and slightly golden. Serve immediately.

RAINBOW FRUIT CUP

My husband's very favorite dessert is a combination of cut-up fruits that are in season. Use fresh, ripe fruits to make your own colorful combinations. A favorite combination of Shelly's is:

1 apple, unpeeled, cut into chunks
1 pear, unpeeled, cut into chunks
1 orange, peeled, sliced
1/2 banana, sliced
1/4 cup freshly squeezed orange juice

Toss fruit together in large glass bowl. Pour juice over mixed fruit and serve well chilled. Note: When melons are in season in the summer, combine them with cut-up plums and peaches for a light dessert. When you are off your diet and maintaining your weight, you can add a bit of shredded coconut and two tablespoons of chopped nuts to your fruit cup for a delicious treat. Yogurt mixed with 1 tablespoon of honey makes a lovely topping for cut-up fruit desserts, as well.

VIENNESE FRUIT COMPOTE

This delicious dessert recipe was given to me by Johanna Roth.

3/4 cup canned peach slices, juice pack
3/4 cup canned pineapple chunks, juice pack
10 large red cherries, sliced
3/4 teaspoon caraway seed
1 teaspoon grated lemon peel
1/2 teaspoon grated orange peel
1/4 teaspoon ground mace
1/8 teaspoon ground allspice
2 tablespoons orange juice

Drain peaches and pineapple and save juices. Mix fruits with cherries in pretty serving bowl. Combine fruit juices in saucepan with caraway, grated peels, spices, and orange juice. Heat to boiling, cover, and simmer for 10 minutes. Cool slightly. Pour over fruit. Cover and chill overnight. Pretty when served in stemmed glasses topped with a dot of yogurt.

The Rainbow

A Poem by Sauci Churchill

We chose this poem by our friend Sauci Churchill to conclude our book because it expresses all the pleasures of eating the full spectrum of nature's colorful foods, and our own best wishes to you as you discover them.

The Rainbow

Soup begins to boil
the pot lid bows
to bay leaf
dances to dill
chive jives
onions are studded
with cloves
the kitchen is a temple
and I high priestess

The mailman
twitches his nose
at my hot broth
turnips tremble
at my touch
carrots rise
at my command
I chop and chop
parsley sways
pots play stove top music

Suddenly a lentil
leaps into the cauldron
black turtle beans
stew in their juices
waiting for the
final consummation

On the street
burglars reach
into their sacks
for silver spoons
I reel with power
pepper fills the air
the room sings hosannas
fire licks the kettle
the door flies open
a rainbow streams
into the kitchen
finds the pot

—*Sauci Churchill*

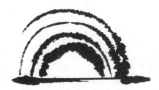

appendix

NATIONAL CANCER INSTITUTE'S "SAVOR THE SPECTRUM— 5 A DAY FOR BETTER HEALTH" PROGRAM

In the Spring of 2002, the National Cancer Institute (NCI)—a component of the U.S. government's National Institute of Health—presented its "Savor the Spectrum" program to promote healthier eating for cancer prevention. You will find the information they provide on the nutritional value of various colored fruits and vegetables supports the concept of our 7-Day Color Diet and gives you a scientific basis for healthy colorful eating. It is reprinted here by permission of the NCI for your further education. Please check their web site for more information on this educational campaign (www.5aday.gov).

A Statement from the National Cancer Institute

We are challenging Americans to go beyond "Sample the Spectrum," by urging them to "Savor the Spectrum" and eat even more colorful fruits and vegetables. By eating red, white, blue, orange, and green fruits and vegetables every day, Americans will not only taste a wide variety of delicious fruits and vegetables but they can improve their health. "Eating the rainbow" provides a mix of phytochemicals which are substances found only in plants that help your body fight off disease and promote good health. Current research shows that phytochemicals from the different color groups are powerful disease-fighters that help protect against cancer, heart disease, cataracts, macular degeneration, and other disease.

Color Your Daily Diet

It's time to get colorful. Color your daily diet with bright oranges (carrots, mandarin oranges, sweet potatoes and mango), deep reds (tomatoes, cherries, and strawberries), dark greens (broccoli, asparagus, and kale), beautiful blues and purples (blueberries, eggplant, and plums), and accent it with sunshine yellow (squash, pineapple, and corn).

"Here's the rule to live by when filling up your plate," advises Gloria Stables, M.S., R.D., director of the NCI Program "Sample the Spectrum." "The more reds, oranges, greens, yellows, and blues you see on the plate, the more health promoting properties you are getting from your fruit and vegetable choices."

As Stables points out, "aesthetics aren't the only reason to eat the rainbow of colors. Nutrition research shows that colorful fruits and vegetables contain essential vitamins, minerals and phytochemicals that help prevent diseases such as cancer, promote health and help you feel great."

Reds

Deep reds and pinks added to your daily diet provide a powerful antioxidant called lycopene. Lycopene, found in tomatoes, red and pink grapefruit, and watermelon reduce the risk of select cancers, including prostate cancer.

Greens

The National Cancer Institute says, "Eat your greens." Green vegetables look great and taste great. They are rich in the phytochemicals that keep us healthy. For example, the carotenoids—lutein and zeaxanthin—are found in spinach, collards, kale, and broccoli have antioxidant properties that protect our eyes by keeping the retina strong. Green vegetables (like cabbage, Brussels sprouts, cauliflower, kale, and turnips) may reduce the risk of cancerous tumors as well.

Oranges

Orange is a must in our daily diet. Orange fruits and vegetables like sweet potatoes, mangos, carrots, and apricots include beta carotene. This carotenoid is a natural antioxidant and enhances our immune system. In addition to being a powerful health-protector, the orange group is rich in Vitamin C and Vitamin E. Folate, usually in leafy greens, is also found in orange fruits and vegetables. As the NCI points out, "With a chemical make-up this good for you, the orange group should always be part of your daily diet."

Yellows

Bright yellows are also high in essential vitamins and carotenoids. Pineapple, for example, is rich with Vitamin C, manganese, and the natural enzyme, bromelain. Bromelain aids in digestion and reduces bloating.

Purples

Purples are full of flavonoids, phytochemicals, and antioxidants.

Anthocyanins, a phytochemical, are pigments responsible for the purple color in fruits and vegetables, and they may help defend against harmful carcinogens. Blueberries, in particular, are rich in Vitamin C and folic acid and high in fiber and potassium.

5 A Day for Better Health

The goal of the National 5 A Day for Better Health Program is to increase the consumption of fruits and vegetables in the United States to 5 to 9 servings every day. In addition to this goal, the program seeks to inform Americans that eating fruits and vegetables can improve their health and reduce the risk of cancer and other diseases, including heart disease, hypertension, diabetes, and macular degeneration. The 5 A Day Program also provides consumers with practical and easy ways to incorporate more fruits and vegetables into their daily eating patterns.

Since its inception in 1991, the 5 A Day for Better Health Program has become one of the most widely recognized health promotion programs in the world. As the largest public/private partnership for nutrition education, the 5 A Day Program's strength is the combined efforts of the National Cancer Institute (NCI), the Produce for Better Health Foundation, the American Cancer Society, the Centers for Disease Control and Prevention, the United States Department of Agriculture, United Fresh Fruit and Vegetable Association, Produce Marketing Association, and the National Alliance for Nutrition and Activity.

Results of the program's efforts have been encouraging. The percentage of Americans who know they should eat 5 or more servings of fruits and vegetables a day has increased nearly fivefold—from 8 to 36 percent—since the program began in 1991. Even better is the fact that during the first three years of the program, the average adult's daily consumption of fruits and vegetables increased significantly. Data from the United States Department of Agriculture's Continuing Surveys of Food Intakes by Individuals (CSFII) shows that in 1989-1991, adults ate an average of 3.9 daily servings of fruits and vegetables. In 1994-1996 that number had increased to approximately 4.6 servings per day—less than half a serving from the recommended minimum of five.

Glossary

Allicin

Allicin, a phytochemical found most notably in onions and garlic, is considered to be protective against cancer and heart disease. Allicin is most widely recognized for its action as an antiviral, antifungal, and antibacterial agent with the ability to block the toxins produced by bacteria and viruses. It is also an antioxidant and helps to eliminate toxins, which is why garlic is sometimes considered a "detoxifier."

Anthocyanins

Anthocyanins represent a group of phytochemicals within the larger category of phytochemicals called "phenolics." Anthocyanins give intense color to certain red and/or blue fruits and vegetables, most notably the blueberry. These plant pigments are very powerful antioxidants and have been studied extensively for their ability to fight heart disease and cancer and to delay several diseases associated with the aging process.

Antioxidant

Antioxidants are found naturally in many fruits and vegetables and act to protect cells from damage caused by the by-products (free radicals) of everyday metabolism and toxic substances in the environment and food. Over time, free radicals can significantly damage cells and lead to a number of diseases associated with aging. Antioxidants act as little vacuum cleaners, eliminating free radicals as they circulate throughout the body, preventing them from doing damage.

Beta Carotene

Beta carotene is a common phytochemical within a group of over 600 called carotenoids. It is found in bright orange-colored fruits and vegetables such as carrots, pumpkins, peaches, and sweet potatoes. In the body, beta carotene is converted to vitamin A, which has many vital functions including the growth and repair of body tissues, formation of bones and teeth, resistance of the body to infection, and development of healthy eye tissues. Whereas vitamin A supplements can be toxic, excess beta carotene is safely stored away and converted to vitamin A only when the body needs it.

Bioflavonoids

Bioflavonoids represent a group of phytochemicals found primarily in citrus fruits. They belong to a large group of more than 2,000 phytochemicals called phenols that are known to be very powerful antioxidants. Bioflavonoids are studied for their ability to delay or prevent some of the effects of the aging process. Bioflavonoids, in particular, have been associated with a decrease in symptoms of arthritis, decreased risk for heart disease and cancer, and lower cholesterol levels.

Indoles

Indoles are a group of phytochemicals that fall within a much larger group called organosulfur compounds. Organosulfur compounds are found in cruciferous vegetables including broccoli, bok choy, cabbage, kale, Brussels sprouts, and turnips. These phytochemicals all contain sulfur, which gives vegetables that contain them a pungent flavor. Each phytochemical within the organosulfur group delivers specific health benefits. Indoles, in particular, are able to bind to cancer-causing chemicals and activate "detox enzymes" that destroy them and prevent damage to cells.

Lutein

Lutein is a phytochemical found most often in leafy green vegetables, but also in other fruits and vegetables. Lutein belongs to a group of over 600 phytochemicals called carotenoids, which are plant pigments that function as antioxidants. Lutein is a component of the macula of the eye, responsible for detailed vision. Evidence suggests that eating foods high in lutein may prevent and slow macular degeneration, a leading cause of blindness in the elderly. As an antioxidant, lutein reduces the amount of free radical damage to the macula and may also help prevent the formation of cataracts, reduce the risk of heart disease, and protect against breast cancer.

Lycopene

Lycopene is one of over 600 phytochemicals called carotenoids with very powerful disease-fighting capabilities, particularly against prostate cancer. Lycopene is associated with the red color in tomatoes. Tomato-based products such as tomato sauce, tomato soup, and tomato juice have the most concentrated source of lycopene. Cooked tomato sauces are associated with greater health benefits, compared to uncooked, because the heating process makes lycopene more easily absorbed by the body. Also, lycopene is fat-soluble, meaning that in order for the body to absorb it, it has to be eaten with at least a small amount of fat. Lycopene has been associated with a reduced risk for many cancers and protection against heart attacks, though research continues on other potential health benefits.

Macular Degeneration

Age-related macular degeneration is the number one cause of severe vision loss or legal blindness in adults over 60 in the U.S. More than one in 10 adults aged 65 to 74, and 28 percent of those 75 years or older have the disease. Age-related macular degeneration reduces "straight ahead" central vision necessary for normal functioning. Risk for macular degeneration increases with age and smoking and dietary factors may also play a role. Certain green leafy vegetables like spinach and kale and brightly colored fruits and vegetables like mangoes, oranges, and cantaloupes contain phyto-chemicals called carotenoids that may reduce the risk for macular degeneration.

Phenolics

Phenolics represent a very large cat-egory of over 2,000 phytochemicals. The term phenol comes from the chemical structure of these phyto-chemicals that vary from having one to several "phenol groups." Phenol groups have the ability to sweep up many free radicals as they circulate through the bloodstream. For this reason, phenolics are considered to be some of the most powerful antioxidants and are studied for their ability to slow down the aging process. However, phenolics also exhibit a wide range of other health benefits, which include anti-inflammatory, anti-allergy, anti-clotting, anti-tumor, and heart protective effects.

Phytochemical

Phytochemicals are defined as sub-stances found only in plants that provide health benefits in addition to those provided by vitamins and minerals alone. Phytochemicals, which represent thousands of differ-ent components in plant foods, differ from vitamins and minerals as they are not considered "essential" nutrients. But, eating an abundance of phytochemicals from various fruits and vegetables has been asso-ciated with the prevention and/or treatment of at least four of the leading causes of death in the U.S.—cancer, heart disease, dia-betes, and high blood pressure. The specific phytochemical content of different fruits and vegetables tends to vary by color and each has unique functions. Some phyto-chemicals act as antioxidants, some protect and regenerate essential nutrients, and others work to de-activate cancer-causing substances.

National Cancer Institute

The National Cancer Institute, a world leader in biomedical cancer research, is the national health authority for the 5 A Day for Better Health Program. NCI provides lead-ership for the program through the implementation of a national media campaign, support of state 5 A Day programs, coordination of national partnership efforts and activities, and funding of nutrition behavior change research.

At the local level, 55 state and U.S. territorial health agencies are licensed by NCI to establish and coordinate 5 A Day programs with-in their states and territories to reach consumers with the 5 A Day message. The national partnership is implemented at the community level through statewide coalitions involving both industry and state licensees. Coalition participants include state and county health agencies, state departments of edu-cation, state departments of agricul-ture, cooperative extensions, volun-tary agencies, businesses, hospitals, and state dietetics associations.

Produce for Better Health Foundation

The Produce for Better Health Foundation serves as the central coordinator for members of industry involved in spreading the 5 A Day message, which includes virtually all segments of the fruit and vegetable industry, including fresh, frozen, dried, canned, and juice.

Contact:

LaTonya Kittles
National Cancer Institute
Phone: 301/451-6055
Kittlesl@mail.nih.gov

Lorelei Di Sogra, EdD, RD
National Cancer Institute
Director, 5 A Day For Better
  Health Program
Phone: 301/496-8520

RECOMMENDED READING

Brody, Jane. *Jane Brody's Good Food Book: Living the High-Carbohydrate Way.* Bantam, 1987.

Jane Brody's Nutrition Book: A Lifetime Guide to Good Eating for Better Health and Weight Control by the Personal Health Columnist of the New York Times. Bantam, 1989.

Jane Brody's Good Food Gourmet: Recipes and Menus for Delicious and Healthful Entertaining. W.W. Norton, 1990.

Jane Brody's Good Seafood Book. Fawcett, 1995.

Jane Brody's Allergy Fighter. Castle, 2000.

The New York Times Guide to Alternative Health. Henry Holt, 2001.

Bruno, Frank I., Ph.D. *Think Yourself Thin.* Nash, 1975.

Burros, Marian. *Pure and Simple.* Morrow, 1982.

Carper, Jean. *The Brand Name Nutrition Counter.* Bantam, 1992.

Cordell, Franklin D., Ph.D., and Gale R. Geibler, Ph.D. *Psychological War on Fat.* Argus, 1995.

Davis, Adelle. *Let's Cook It Right.* Harcourt Brace Jovanovich, 1987.

Deutsch, Ronald M. *Realities of Nutrition.* Bell, 1993.

Glen, Morton B., M.D. *But I Don't Eat That Much.* Dutton, 1974.

Godfrey, Bronwen, Carol Flinders, and Laurel Robertson. *Laurel's Kitchen: A Handbook for Vegetarian Cookery and Nutrition.* Nilgiri, 1986.

Heber, David, M.D. *What Color Is Your Diet?* Regan Books, 2000.

Hewitt, Jean. *The New York Times Natural Foods Cookbook.* Avon, 1989.

Jordan, Henry A., M.D., Leonard S. Levitz, Ph.D., and Gordon M. Kimbrell, Ph.D. *Eating Is O.K.* Rawson, 1989.

Joseph, James, M.D. *The Color Code.* Hyperion, 2002.

Meyers, Perla. *The Seasonal Kitchen: A Return to Fresh Foods.* Vintage Books, 1989.

Ornish, Dean. *Eat More, Weigh Less.* Quill, 2000.

Sears, Barry, Ph.D. *The Soy Zone.* Regan Books, 2000.

Stuart, Richard B., Ph.D. *Act Thin, Stay Thin.* Norton, 1987.

index